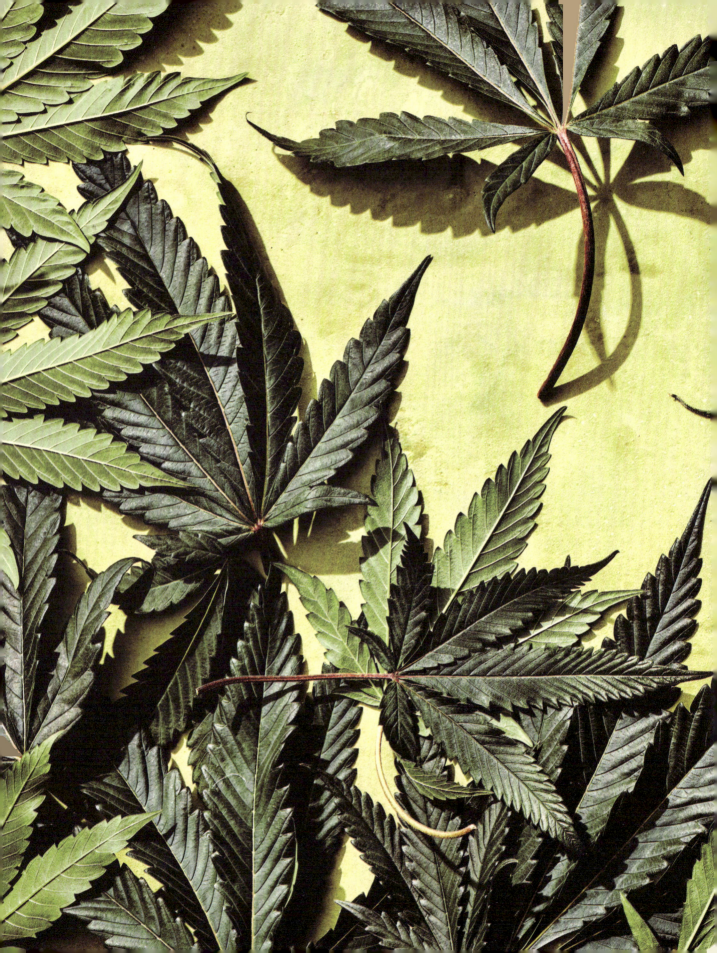

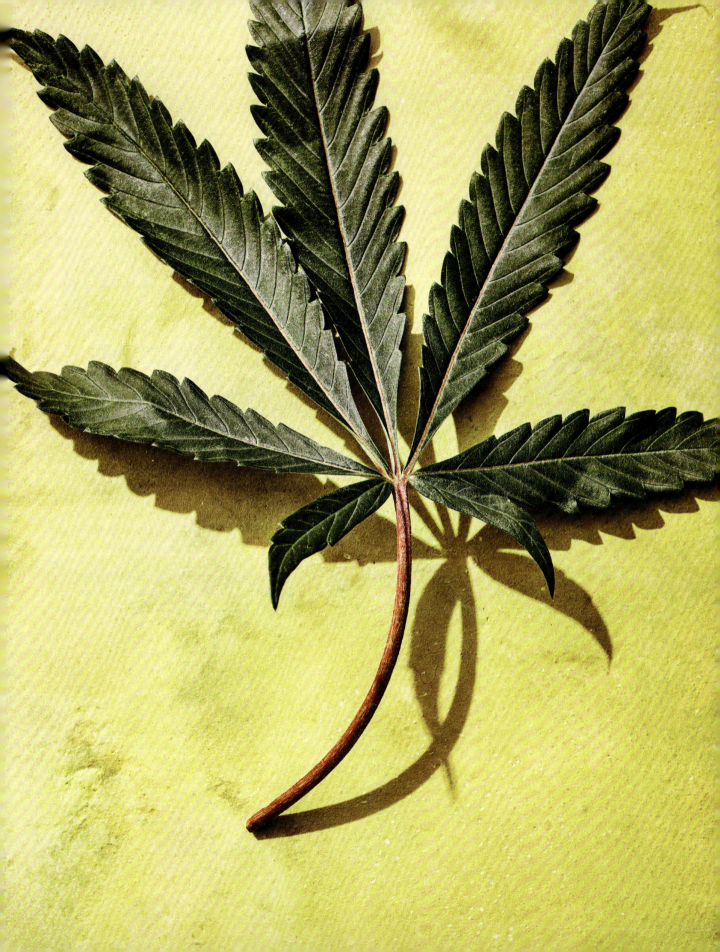

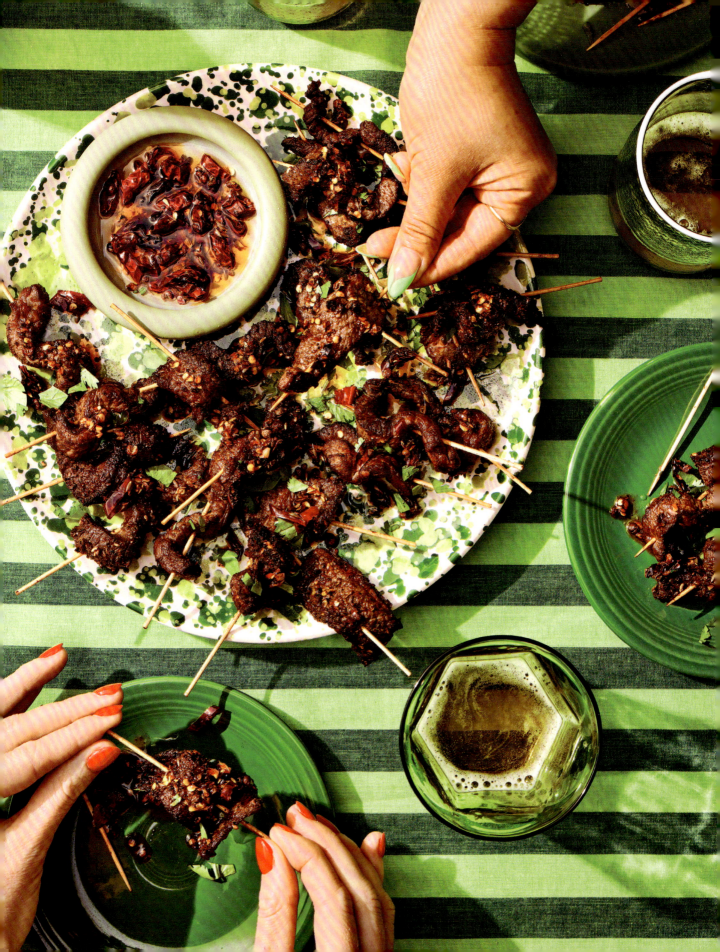

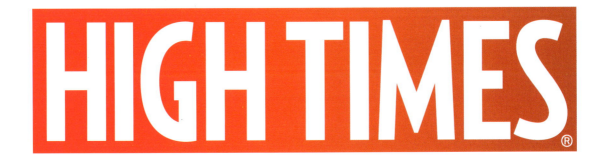

LET'S GET BAKED!

THE OFFICIAL
CANNABIS COOKBOOK

Blazingly Good Recipes to Satisfy Your Every Craving

Haejin Chun 🍁 Jamie Evans

Photography by Eva Kolenko

SAN RAFAEL · LOS ANGELES · LONDON

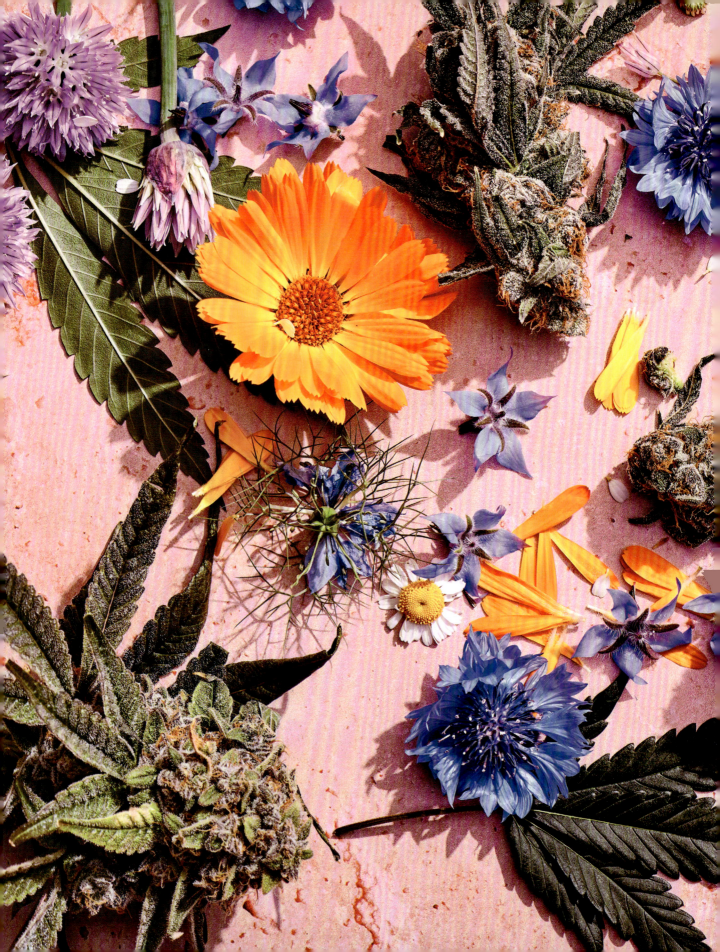

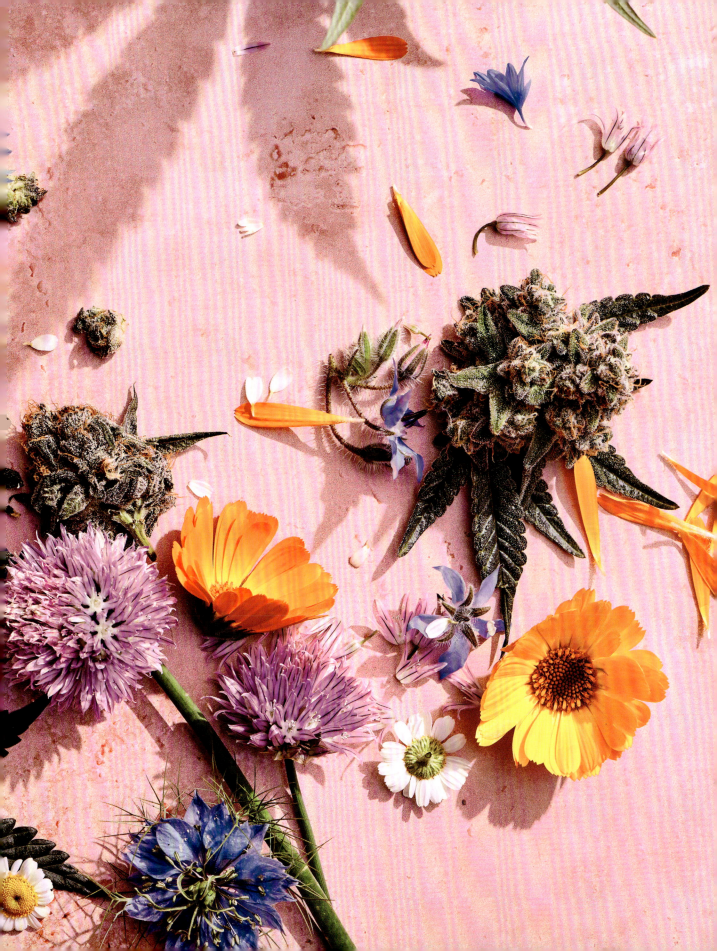

CONTENTS

Introduction 9
Cannabis 101 10

CHAPTER 1:
CANNABIS COOKING ESSENTIALS 13

The Basics 14
Working with Phytocannabinoids & Terpenes 17
A Deep Dive into Decarboxylation 20
Dosage Guide 24
How to Safely Serve Infused Foods & Beverages 28

CHAPTER 2:
THE ART OF COOKING WITH CANNABIS 31

Combining Cannabis with Food 32
Creating Infusions 101 40
Cannabis-Infused Oils 44
Cannabis-Infused Chili Oil 47
Cannabis-Infused Butter 48
Cannabis-Infused Saturated Fats 49
Cannabis-Infused Honey 50
Cannabis-Infused Sugar 51
How to Make Hash-Infused Peanut Oil & Peanut Butter 52
Cannabis-Infused Bitters 56
Cannabis-Infused Alcohol Tincture 58
Cannabis-Infused Simple Syrup 60
Cannabis-Infused Coconut Milk 62
Cannabis-Infused Fruit Syrup 64
Fat-Washed Infusions Two Ways 68

CHAPTER 3:
THE RECIPES

+ **Baked Sweets 72**

Guava Cream Cheese Pastry with Salted Egg Yolk 73
Baked Pears 74
Black Sesame Blondie 77
Mini Blueberry Cheesecake Bites 78
Honey Furikake Cashews 79
Jasmine & Condensed Milk Sandwich Cookies 80
Miso Crème Brûlée 85
Strawberry Matcha Shortcake Cups 86

+ **Baked Savory 88**

Delicata Squash with Goat Cheese & Honey 89
Bulgogi Bbang Puff Pastry 90
Cheesy Kimchi & Tomato Dip 92
Gochujang Dungeness Crab Pot Pie 95
Steamed Egg + Shiitake + Chili Oil 98
Jalapeño Chive Cornbread 99
Miso Ginger Glazed Black Cod 100

+ **No-Bake & Infused Treats 102**
    Lychee Sorbet 103
    Dulce de Leche Peach Toast 104
    Choco Pie Milkshake 106
    Milk Tea-Ramisu 107
    Mango Coconut Tapioca Pudding 109
    Sweet Corn Ice Cream 110
    Tofu Chocolate Pudding 111
    Ooey Gooey Banana Doughnuts with Pandan Condensed Milk 112

+ **Savory Eats 114**
    Chili Garlic Shrimp 115
    Big Bad Fried Chicken 116
    Braised Short Ribs 117
    Juiced Canna Leaf Dumplings 119
    Kabocha Pumpkin Jook with Mochi 123
    Korean Veggie Pancakes 124
    Quick Kimchi Cotton Candy Grapes 125

+ **Cannabis Drinks 126**
    Passion Fruit Canna-Colada 127
    Ginger Peach Creamsicle Smoothie 128
    Peanut Butter Hot Chocolate 129
    Blood Orange Raspberry Sour 130
    Brown Butter Old Fashioned 134
    Detox Juice 137
    Serrano Pineapple Margarita 139
    Shiso Mojito 140
    Watermelon Mint Lemonade 141
    The Dankest Over-the-Top Kimchi Bloody Mary 142

+ **Noninfused Munchies 146**
    Candied Fruit 147
    Carrot Cake Truffles 148
    Cornflake Miso Pressé 151
    Fried Cassava Fries 152
    Grilled Cheese with Caramelized Onions 154
    Mini Korean Corn Dogs 155
    Salvadoran Pupusas 156
    Sichuan Toothpick Lamb 160
    Candied Sweet Potatoes 162
    Chocolate Milk Tea Popsicle 163
    Strawberries and Cream Pavlova 164
    Strawberry White Rabbit Crispy Rice Treats 167

+ **Resources & Works Cited 169**
+ **About the Authors 170**
+ **Acknowledgments 172**

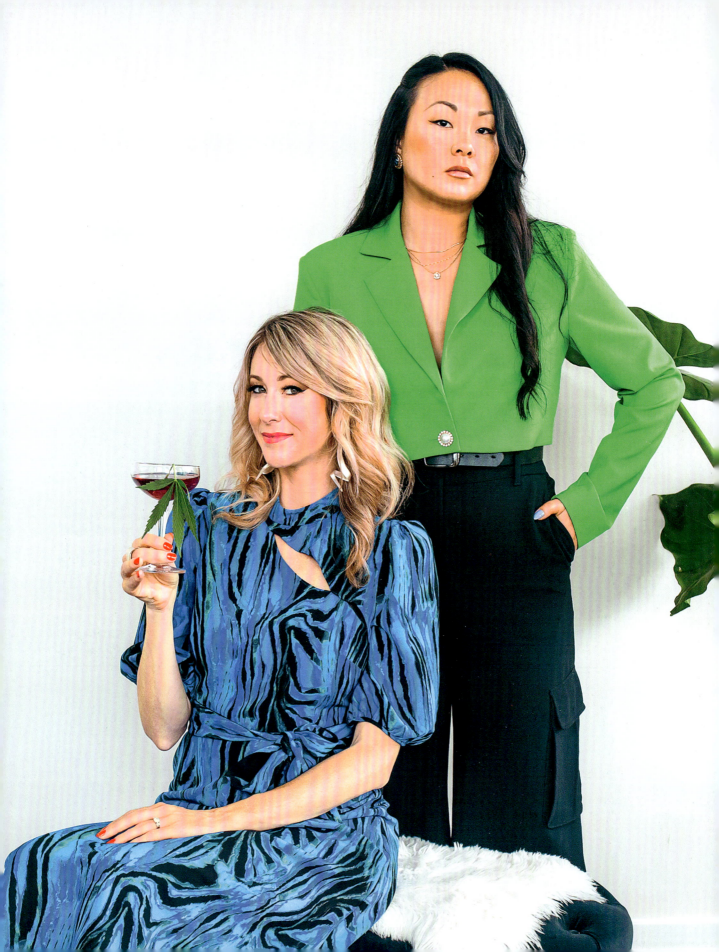

INTRODUCTION

Cooking with cannabis is our passion and personal obsession. There's something so special about working with the plant and witnessing how it brings together people from all walks of life over a heartfelt, comforting meal. The universal language of breaking bread together, combined with the ritual and ceremony of cannabis, is communal alchemy. As culinary cannabis enthusiasts, we believe that cannabis is something to be shared, whether it's at the dinner table, as part of an intimate gathering among friends, or during a celebration. We see cannabis as any other ingredient in the kitchen to work with, but with a little more magic added due to its elevating properties and vast array of aromas and flavors. Cannabis can be incorporated into food and beverages in so many ways, which makes it one of the most exciting ingredients to create with!

Before you embark on this epicurean cannabis journey, we want to quickly introduce ourselves. As you flip through the pages of this book, you'll come across food recipes crafted by Chef Haejin Chun, renowned first-generation Korean American chef, entrepreneur, and founder of the culinary cannabis events company Big Bad Wolf SF. You'll also enjoy a collection of infusions and infused beverage recipes developed by celebrated cannabis cookbook author, cannabis drink expert, and certified sommelier Jamie Evans (also known as The Herb Somm) to keep you high and hydrated. We are both advocating for the destigmatization of cannabis through the culinary arts.

When we were asked to write this cookbook, the stars truly aligned. It was the perfect opportunity to collaborate, celebrate our ethos for cannabis and community, and prepare delicious food and drinks as a love language for the people we share them with. Cannabis is more than just a lifestyle. It is a huge part of who we are, which we express through the recipes in this book—or as we like to say, the *high flavors* we've conceptualized from our cannabis kitchens.

Our passion for cannabis led us to this partnership with High Times, one of the most iconic and influential cannabis platforms in the world. Our mission for this project is not only to share these delicious eats and drinks, but also to provide a little bit of education to help end misconceptions about the cannabis plant, something we collectively believe is crucial to breaking stigmas and having a positive impact on the community and culture.

Knowing this, if you're looking to take your baking and cooking skills to the next level, you've come to the right place! It is an honor to guide you through this journey of learning how to work with cannabis in the kitchen.

Baking and cooking with weed can seem overwhelming at first, but don't worry! We've written this book for beginners and experts alike. But before we get to the actual cooking, it's crucial to understand some of the basics about the cannabis plant itself. Here's a quick overview of how cannabis works with our internal systems and what to expect after consuming cannabis-infused food and beverages. If you're already familiar with this information, feel free to flip to Chapter 1, on page 13.

CANNABIS 101

Cannabis is a miraculous plant, consisting of hundreds of different organic compounds that work together to produce therapeutic effects that impact the mind and body. These compounds are what makes cannabis so unique: The plant naturally produces a myriad of special molecules, including *phytocannabinoids*.

A phytocannabinoid is a cannabinoid or group of chemically similar compounds that are synthesized by plants, such as cannabidiol (CBD) or tetrahydrocannabinol (THC). When consumed, these compounds directly interact with our internal endocannabinoid system (also known as the ECS), delivering enhanced effects.

Although phytocannabinoids can be isolated and consumed on their own, scientists have discovered that the greatest benefits are produced when cannabinoids are combined with organic compounds known as terpenoids (terpenes) and flavonoids, which are also naturally produced by the cannabis plant. When consumed, this powerful blend works in harmony or acts as a beneficial entourage, interacting with cannabinoid receptors in the body. This phenomenon, known as the entourage effect, was discovered in 1998 by Professor Raphael Mechoulam and Professor Shimon Ben-Shabat. Since then, the entourage effect has played an important role in cannabis research and has helped us better understand both how cannabis works with the endocannabinoid system and why consuming full-spectrum cannabis is the best option.

Both humans and mammals have endocannabinoid systems that consist of various endocannabinoids, cannabinoid receptors, and enzymes that are dispersed throughout the body. Miraculously, phytocannabinoids such as THC and CBD are able to stimulate these different receptor sites, helping maintain homeostasis (or your body's happy place).

In addition to CBD and THC, cannabis contains more than one hundred unique phytocannabinoids, each offering different benefits and characteristics that interact with the ECS. For example, tetrahydrocannabivarin (THCV) is potentially a great option for people seeking weight loss because it suppresses the appetite. Similarly, cannabinol (CBN) works wonders for sleep. The good news is we are learning more about these lesser-known phytocannabinoids, which could potentially offer a better solution for targeted healing. Flip to page 17 for an overview of the most common types you might come across at the time we're writing this book.

Smokeables vs. Edibles

Understanding the differences between smoking and eating or drinking cannabis is crucial if you are planning on baking with weed. For starters, smoking cannabis will not produce the same side effects as ingesting it. Knowing this, if you have a high tolerance for smokables, this does not guarantee you'll have a high tolerance for edibles or drinkables, which is largely due to how the body metabolizes phytocannabinoids, namely THC.

When smoked or vaporized, cannabis passes through the lungs before entering the bloodstream. Smokeables tend to have a much higher bioavailability rate (the degree and rate at which a substance is absorbed into the bloodstream) than edibles because phytocannabinoids don't pass through the stomach to the liver. Because of this, the effects of delta-9 THC typically kick in as fast as 30 to 90 seconds; depending on the person and how much was inhaled, the high can last between 1 to 2 hours. In most instances, the effects of vaporized or smoked cannabis come quicker and diminish faster than when eating or drinking THC-infused products.

On the flip side, when eaten, cannabis passes through the stomach and metabolizes in the liver, which converts delta-9 THC to 11-hydroxy-THC (11-hydroxy-delta 9-tetrahydrocannabinol). If you are new to 11-hydroxy-THC, it is a metabolic derivative of THC and an entirely different compound that's formed by the human body when delta-9 THC is metabolized. Unlike delta-9 THC, 11-hydroxy-THC does not naturally occur in the cannabis plant. Once formed, it causes a longer-lasting, more intense high.

> *Tip!* **As you will learn throughout this book, when it comes to eating and drinking cannabis, always follow the golden rule: Start low and go slow. Consume a low number of milligrams, and consume slowly and with intention. With homemade edibles or drinkables, the effects can take as long as 1 to 2 hours to kick in after consumption. It's incredibly important to be patient anytime you're enjoying cannabis-infused food or drinks. If you consume too much at first, the experience can be very uncomfortable—and depending on how much you eat or drink, the high can last eight hours or more. Homemade edibles and drinkables generally take longer to set in, whereas commercially made edibles and drinkables (the cannabis products you'll find at a licensed dispensary) can produce much faster effects, sometimes acting as quickly as 10 to 15 minutes after consumption, depending on how the product was produced. If you want something fast acting, be sure to do your research and consult with a trusted budtender to find a product that works best for your personal needs.**

Let's Get Baked!

Whether you're looking to create some delicious baked sweets, savory eats, cannabis-infused drinks, or noninfused munchies, this cookbook has it all. Throughout each chapter, you will learn important techniques to set you up for success in the kitchen. You begin your cannabis cooking journey in Chapter 1, where you learn key cannabis cooking essentials. Once you've mastered these methods, head to Chapter 2 to discover how to best combine cannabis with food and take a deep dive into making cannabis-infused pantry items at home. Finally, put your skills to the test in Chapter 3 as you create some of our favorite food and drink recipes. From discovering how to properly decarboxylate cannabis flower and concentrates, to learning the art of cooking with cannabis, we encourage you to use this book as your guide through each important process.

While flipping through the pages, you will also discover some unique highlights along the way, such as how to match cannabis with different flavors, tips for choosing the best cannabis products, a chef's checklist before getting started, plus how to make a collection of the tastiest noninfused munchies from some of our favorite culinary cannabis creators!

In addition, this cookbook features a selection of the most celebrated Korean-inspired food recipes by Chef Haejin (a.k.a. Big Bad Wolf), both spinoffs of traditional family recipes and concoctions that reflect her upbringing as a first-generation Korean American growing up in California. You'll also enjoy a collection of some new drink recipes from Jamie (a.k.a. The Herb Somm), so we hope you've come with both a big appetite and a thirst to learn more!

We welcome you to *High Times: The Official Cannabis Cookbook*. Let's get baked!

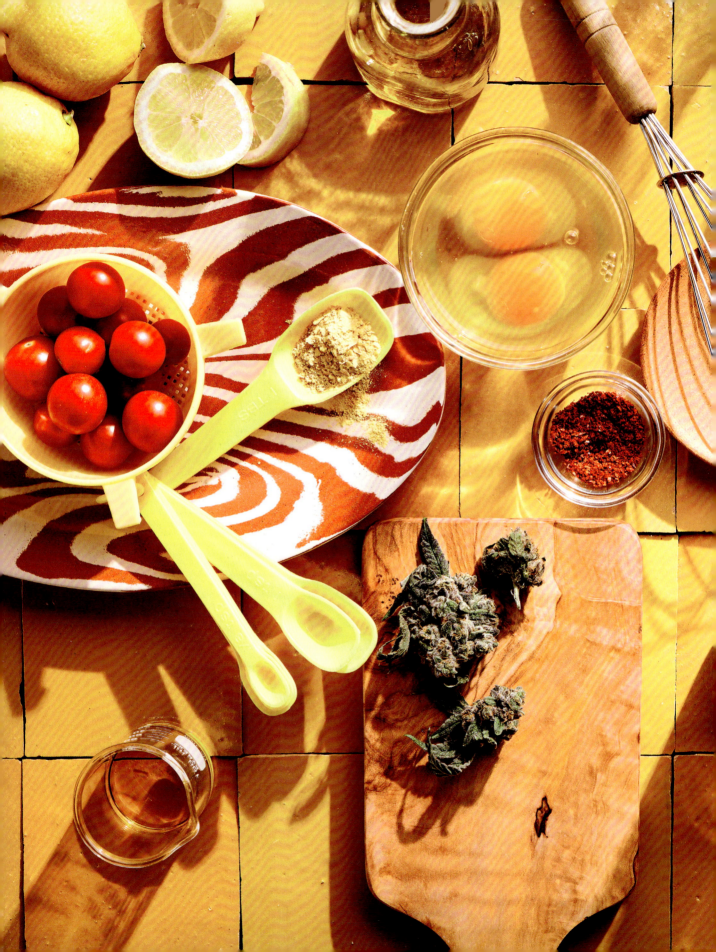

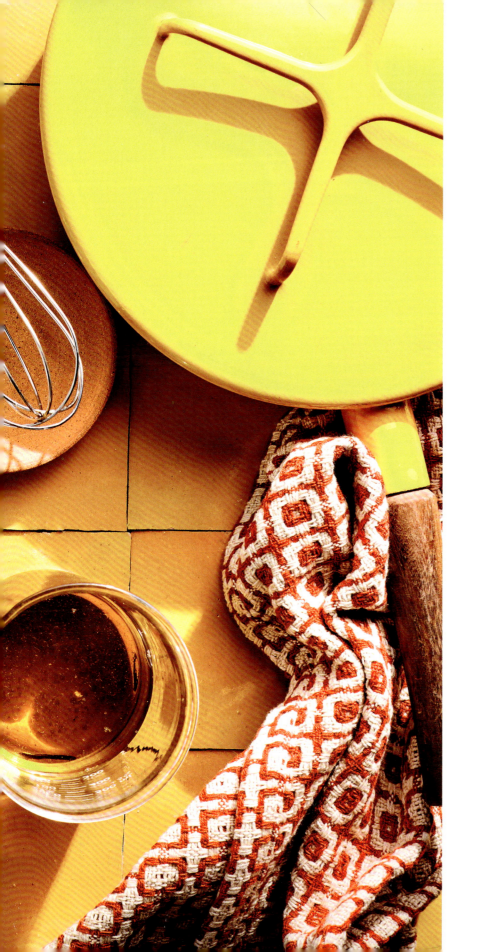

CANNABIS COOKING ESSENTIALS

CHAPTER 1

Considered both an art and a science, learning to properly cook with cannabis is an essential step to creating the best infused recipes. Although it might seem intimidating at first, once you learn the basics, you'll be able to confidently enhance your favorite foods and beverages in the comfort of your kitchen.

Before you start creating your first infused recipe, it's important to familiarize yourself with the basic concepts and methods for cooking with cannabis. In this chapter, you'll learn everything you need to get started, plus more. Consider this your crash course in cannabis cooking essentials. Let's get started!

THE BASICS

If this is your first time using weed as an ingredient, don't worry! By following these step-by-step guidelines, you'll be creating flavorful infused items in no time. To help you master the art of baking with cannabis (some of these topics will also be continued in Chapter 2), here are six essential steps to keep in mind as you get started.

> *Tip!* **If this isn't your first time cooking with herbal products and you have experience working with cannabis as a food or beverage ingredient, jump ahead to page 44 for the infusion recipes.**

1. Select Your Cannabis Ingredient

The first step to cooking with cannabis is selecting what type of cannabis product to use in your recipes. Consider it your base ingredient to be incorporated into oil, butter, simple syrup, tinctures, and more. As you will learn in Chapter 2, you can use many different types of products, depending on your personal needs and what you have access to: cannabis flower, concentrates, isolates, tinctures, and commercially made gourmet cannabis pantry items. Once you choose a product that's right for you, be sure to note the cannabinoid percentages that are listed on the packaging. These numbers are directly related to how strong your infusion will be. Flip to page 32 for more tips on how to select the best cannabis ingredients.

2. Decarboxylate to Activate Your Cannabis

To maximize the yield and create the most potent infusions, decarboxylating (or decarbing) cannabis is a heating method that activates phytocannabinoids. During this process, heat triggers a chemical reaction that releases the carboxylic acids from THCA and CBDA, converting them into THC and CBD to produce more enhanced and intense effects. As you will learn, you can use many methods for decarboxylating cannabis flower and concentrates, ranging in temperatures and techniques. Turn to page 20 for a deep dive into decarboxylation and the best methods to use when decarbing at home.

3. Calculate the Dosage Before Cooking

When cooking with cannabis, calculating the dosage of your infusions is one of the most important steps, especially when working with THC. This simple math to estimate the amount of phytocannabinoids per serving will help you avoid many pitfalls, including overserving yourself or a guest. To calculate this amount properly, flip to page 25 for the formula and page 26 for our recommended dosage guide.

4. Prepare Your Infusion

Now it's time to prepare an infusion to be incorporated into a number of recipes! You can think of these items as infused pantry items; by definition, they are classified as any fat-based or alcohol-based ingredient that has been infused with cannabis. Creating infusions is one of the best ways to integrate THC, CBD, and other cannabis components into food and drinks because you're extracting the organic compounds from the plant using solvents such as butter, chili oil, olive oil, and ethanol. These infused fat-based and alcohol-based ingredients blend seamlessly with your other ingredients and taste delicious. Much like decarboxylated cannabis, you have many methods available for creating infusions, and we explore them in detail. Head to Chapter 2, on page 31, to learn more.

5. Prepare the Recipe

With a stocked cannabis pantry, you are now ready to incorporate your homemade infusions into everyday recipes. Since you'll primarily be using infused oils, butter, honey, and sugar, it's easy to swap noninfused traditional ingredients with these enhanced versions. Just be sure to calculate the estimated dose per serving based on how much you're using, and always use measuring spoons, cups, or calibrated droppers for precise dosing. If you prefer a lower dose, you can also combine noninfused ingredients with the infused versions, if needed (for example, combine 2 teaspoons noninfused traditional butter with 1 teaspoon cannabis-infused butter to equal 1 tablespoon total). Throughout this book, you will find a number of delicious recipes with recommended dosages, but feel free to customize them based on your personal preferences and needs. Just be sure that the ingredient ratios remain the same so that the recipe is prepared correctly. Turn to Chapter 3, on page 71, to get cooking.

6. Enjoy Edibles Responsibly

After preparing your cannabis-infused food and beverages, the final step is learning how to enjoy them safely and responsibly. Pay close attention to how much THC you've consumed, and remember to be patient. It can take 1 to 2 hours for homemade edibles and drinkables to kick in, so don't eat more just because you're not feeling anything right away. Remember the golden rule: *Start low and go slow*. Flip to page 28 for more tips and tricks on safely preparing and serving cannabis-infused cuisine at home.

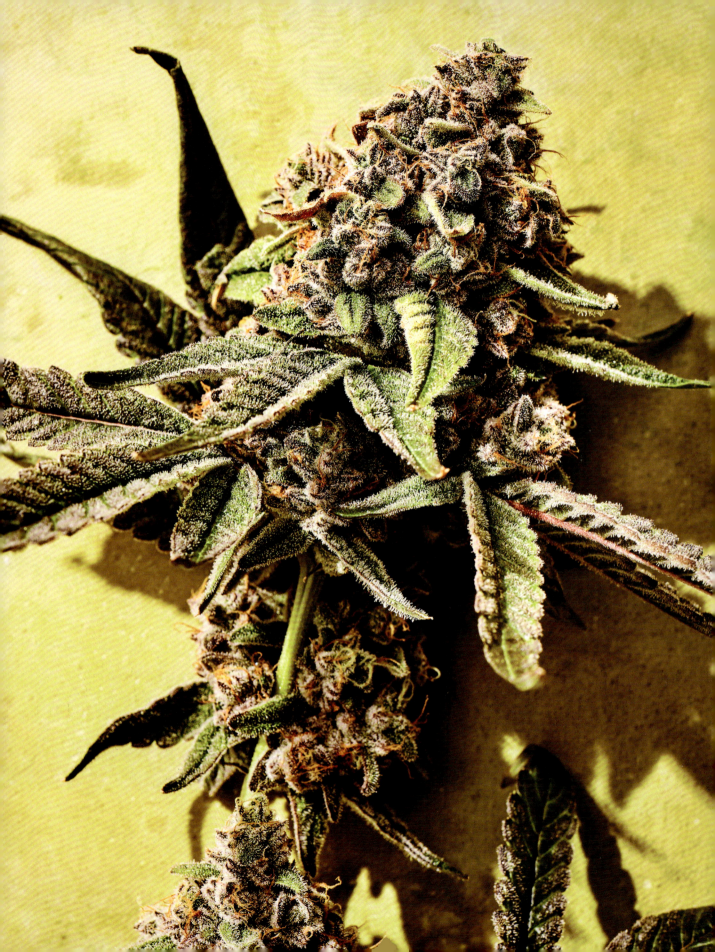

WORKING WITH PHYTOCANNABINOIDS & TERPENES

Unlike other ingredients, cannabis is a unique plant to cook with because it contains varying levels of phytocannabinoids and terpenes (refer to page 10 for an introduction to these terms). THC and CBD are the most widely known phytocannabinoids, but researchers have discovered more than 100 different cannabinoid compounds and more than 200 terpenes in cannabis so far. Although only a handful are present in high enough amounts to deliver noticeable effects, it's important to familiarize yourself with the most common types as you begin to work with cannabis.

Most Common Phytocannabinoids

As you've learned, phytocannabinoids are a group of organic plant compounds that are synthesized by cannabis. When consumed, these powerful compounds directly interact with our internal endocannabinoid systems, delivering therapeutic effects. Here are the most common phytocannabinoid compounds you'll most likely come across:

CBD (CANNABIDIOL): A great place to start if you're a beginner. CBD does not produce the same sense of euphoria or mind-altering effects as THC, but it is indeed psychoactive because it interacts with the brain to help reduce anxiety and relieve stress. As a nonintoxicating cannabinoid, CBD is also a powerful anti-inflammatory and acts as an antioxidant.

CBDA (CANNABIDIOLIC ACID): The acid form of CBD that's created by CBGA. CBDA produces anti-inflammatory and antianxiety effects similar to CBD, but it does not interact with the typical elements of the endocannabinoid system. When exposed to heat, CBDA converts to CBD via decarboxylation.

CBG (CANNABIGEROL): A nonintoxicating cannabinoid that's present in small quantities in most strains. Originating as CBGA (also known as the mother of all cannabinoids), the acidic form of CBG is the precursor for developing THC and CBD. Difficult to extract, CBG acts as an antianxiety, anti-inflammatory, and antibacterial, among other positive side effects.

CBN (CANNABINOL): Mildly intoxicating, CBN is best known for its sedative and pain-relieving side effects. This sleepy cannabinoid is produced by the oxidation of THC and degradation from light and heat after the cannabis is harvested.

DELTA-8 THC (DELTA-8 TETRAHYDROCANNABINOL): Causes similar effects to delta-9 THC (the most recognized form of THC) but is much less potent. Binding to the endocannabinoid system, delta-8 THC will get you high, and it presents feelings of euphoria, sedation, and relief. Compared to delta-9, delta-8 can be a milder experience. Just be sure to obtain your products from a reputable source!

DELTA-9 THC (DELTA-9 TETRAHYDROCANNABINOL): The THC we typically think of when we hear the term. This cannabinoid is the primary intoxicating component of cannabis that's found in several variations. Directly binding to CB1 and CB2 receptors in the brain, delta-9 THC delivers a variety of therapeutic benefits, including pain relief, nausea mediation, anti-inflammatory benefits, and much more. Be patient when experimenting with this powerful cannabinoid—it will get you high! Consuming too much THC can result in some negative side effects, such as anxiety, dizziness, and paranoia.

THCA (TETRAHYDROCANNABINOLIC ACID): The most prominent compound found in raw cannabis and the nonintoxicating acid form of THC. When THCA is exposed to heat, it converts to THC via decarboxylation. Knowing this, it's best to keep THCA products away from heat if you want to enjoy this phytocannabinoid in its nonintoxicating form. This cannabinoid is a powerful anti-inflammatory and pain reliever without the euphoric attributes of THC.

THCV (TETRAHYDROCANNABIVARIN): Presenting some intoxicating effects, THCV is a variation of THC that is known to suppress the appetite. Due to its interaction with CB1 receptors in the brain, THCV reduces feelings that trigger hunger, which makes it useful for weight loss. THCV can also deliver some uplifting feelings, almost like drinking a cup of coffee.

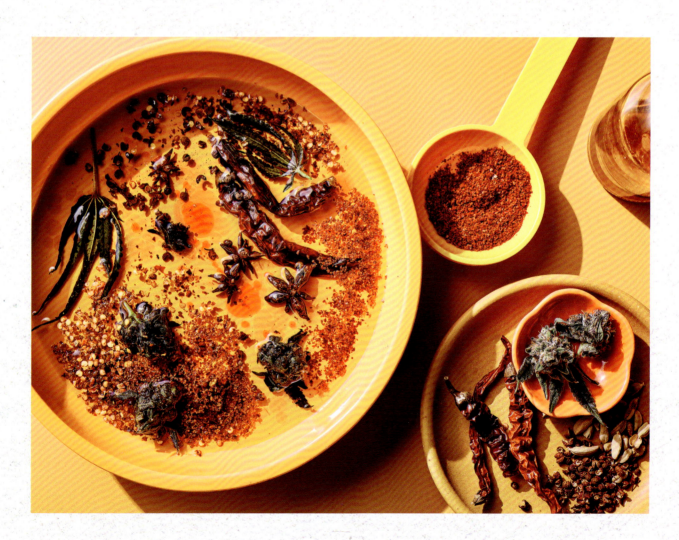

Most Common Terpenes

Found in many herbs, spices, fruits, and flowers, terpenes are naturally occurring organic compounds that deliver unique aromas, flavors, and therapeutic properties. In cannabis, terpenes are what makes different strains smell and taste a certain way. They work in tandem with phytocannabinoids to deliver enhanced effects. You can also pair cannabis terpenes with the other ingredients in your recipes to create the best flavor matches. Here are the some of the most common terpenes to familiarize yourself with:

BETA-CARYOPHYLLENE: One of the most common terpenes found in cannabis, this terpene displays recognizable notes of cinnamon, black pepper, clove, and copaiba. Studies have shown that it acts as an anti-inflammatory, antioxidant, antianxiety, and pain relief option. Beta-caryophyllene is also calming, promoting a stress-free demeanor.

HUMULENE: Also found in hops, humulene is a euphoric, relaxing, and sedative terpene that presents earthy aromas and flavors of hops, fresh-cut wood, coriander, and cloves. It's best known for its anti-inflammatory, antibacterial, and pain-relieving effects.

LIMONENE: If you're a fan of citrus, you're a fan of limonene. This terpene displays pronounced lemon, lime, grapefruit, and tangerine notes. Limonene is best known to enhance moods, but it also acts as a natural stress reducer, promotes weight loss, and fights depression.

LINALOOL: Found in lavender, citrus, and a variety of other flowers, this terpene promotes relaxation and sleep. Both tranquil and restorative, linalool is associated with the floral notes of cannabis, displaying aromas and flavors of lavender, citrus blossom, violet, and rose. It also acts as an antifungal, antidepressant, and potential sleep aid.

MYRCENE: One of the most prevalent terpenes found in cannabis, myrcene is often characterized by its earthy and dank notes of mixed herbs, forest floor, mushroom, skunk, and overripe tropical fruits such as mango. Studies have shown this terpene has the ability to relax muscles, slow bacterial growth, and promote sleep. It is known to be a sedative, so it's recommended to enjoy myrcene-rich strains before bedtime.

PINENE: This refreshing terpene is most commonly associated with pine trees and other cone-bearing seed plants; however, high levels of pinene can also be found in cannabis, dill, rosemary, pine needles, pine nuts, and other herbs. In cannabis, you'll come across *alpha-pinene* and *beta-pinene*, which act as an anti-inflammatory, can help with asthma, promote alertness, provide energy, and aid in memory retention. You'll stay alert and focused with pinene-rich strains.

When baking and cooking, preserving these precious compounds must be top of mind because they are the driving force behind the flavor and effect of the infusions you create. Both phytocannabinoids and terpenes are extremely sensitive to heat, so it's imperative to keep cooking temperatures as low as possible, to prevent loss. Flip to page 22 for the Baking & Cooking Temperature Guide to assist you as you begin cooking with cannabis.

A DEEP DIVE INTO DECARBOXYLATION

To unlock the full potential of your cannabis infusions, decarboxylation is a recommended heating technique that activates CBD and THC. Many approaches to decarbing cannabis flower and concentrates exist, so here are the most common methods used to create the dankest infusions.

THE OVEN METHOD

The most common method when decarbing at home is to use the oven to activate your cannabis flower and concentrates. Exposing cannabis to heat between 240°F and 295°F (115°C and 146°C) for 20 to 60 minutes converts THCA to THC and also converts CBDA to CBD. As a rule, you want to heat for a shorter time at higher temperatures or for a longer time at lower temperatures between this range, which is considered the most general heat range for decarbing. However, temperatures can fluctuate based on the product you're using and the effect you're trying to achieve. For example, to best preserve cannabinoids and terpenes in cannabis flower, you can decarb at 230°F (110°C). Just be aware that not all the THCA may convert to THC. Depending on your oven, it might take some experimentation to see what works best for you.

> *Tip!* When using the oven method, be aware that your kitchen will be filled with a very strong cannabis aroma. If you're worried about disturbing your neighbors or a landlord, it's best to use a different method, such as a decarboxylation device or sous vide, both available online.

How to Properly Decarboxylate Flower

To decarboxylate cannabis flower, we recommend decarbing at lower temperatures. Preheat your oven to 240°F (115°C). As your oven is heating, line a baking sheet with parchment paper or aluminum foil. Wearing gloves, use your fingers (or scissors) to break up the cannabis flower into pea-size pieces; then evenly spread the pieces over the baking sheet. When the oven is heated, simply put the baking sheet in the oven and bake for 20 to 30 minutes. Remove from heat, let cool, and store in an airtight sealed mason jar until you're ready to use. If you plan on using flower, be sure to use all parts of the flower, including buds, stems, and shake—just use the same strain so you can calculate the dosage accurately.

> *Tip!* When breaking up your flower for decarboxylation, do not use a grinder. It disrupts your phytocannabinoids and terpenes, making it difficult to decarb properly. Instead, simply use your fingers or scissors to break up the buds into smaller pieces, and then proceed as directed.

Activation Temperatures for Decarboxylation

Phytocannabinoids	°F	°C
THCA*	240-275	115-135
CBDA**	240-295	115-146

*Converts from THCA to THC if you heat between 240°F and 275°F (115°C and 135°C) for 20 minutes to 1 hour

**Converts from CBDA to CBD if you heat between 240°F and 295°F (115°C and 146°C) for 20 minutes to 1 hour

***Sourced from *Cannabis Drinks: Secrets to Crafting CBD and THC Beverages at Home*

How to Properly Decarboxylate Concentrates

To preserve the quality of concentrates, it's recommended to decarboxylate at lower temperatures. For best results, decarb between 200°F and 240°F (93°C to 115°C), depending on the product you're working with. As the oven preheats, transfer the concentrate into a small oven-safe glass baking dish. Be sure to use a clear glass dish so you can keep an eye on the concentrate during the heating process. Cover the baking dish with a lid or aluminum foil to prevent excess evaporation, and then place it in the oven. Once your concentrate has completely liquified and is consistent, it's decarboxylated. If you want to go the extra mile, you can use a thermometer to check the internal temperature. Just remember to keep temperatures low so you don't burn off any precious cannabis compounds.

DECARBOXYLATION DEVICE

One of the best ways to accurately and evenly decarboxylate cannabis is to use a device that has been designed specifically for decarboxylation. Although several options are available at the time we're writing this book, we highly recommend investing in the Ardent FX All-In-One Decarboxylation and Infusion device. With a push of a button, you can decarb, infuse, and bake, all in the same device. It's easy to use and incredibly precise because it fully converts almost 100 percent of the THC in your flower (although it does take longer than the oven method and requires additional cool-down time). Decarb devices are also much more discreet than the oven method when it comes to dank smells and cleanup.

SOUS VIDE

For those looking for a fragrance-free option, using a sous vide machine to decarboxylate is another discrete and beginner-friendly way to activate cannabis because it allows for precise, even heating. If you're using flower, Monica Lo, sous vide expert and creator of the popular cannabis blog Sous Weed, recommends breaking up the cannabis into pea-size pieces and adding it to a freezer-safe zip seal bag or vacuum seal zip bag specially made for sous vide. If you don't have a vacuum sealer, you can manually press out the air; however, for best results, a vacuum seal guarantees even heating. Submerge the bag underwater at 194°F (90°C) for 2 hours; you may need to use tongs or sous vide magnets to keep the bag submerged as it may release gas and cause the bag to float. Use tongs to remove, and let cool before opening the bag. Because of the low decarb temperature, this heating technique best captures terpene profiles. The whole process does take longer, but one of the other perks is the ability to set and forget. For multitaskers, this method also frees up your oven if you need to work on other dishes while you wait for your infusion.

WHEN NOT TO DECARBOXYLATE

Although decarboxylation is the most common method used when cooking with cannabis, sometimes you should avoid it. If you want to consume THCA or CBDA, keep your cannabis products away from heat. To access these phytocannabinoids, we recommend juicing raw cannabis leaves or adding fresh cannabis flower (not decarboxylated) directly to ethanol to make an alcohol-based tincture. For the best extraction, use a clear, unflavored, high-proof grain alcohol (beginning at 120 proof or higher). By avoiding decarboxylation, you'll also best preserve terpene profiles. Flip to page 40 for more tips on how to create tinctures at home.

BAKING & COOKING TEMPERATURE GUIDE

To best preserve your phytocannabinoids and terpenes and also avoid degradation, don't exceed the following temperatures when baking or cooking with cannabis.

Phytocannabinoids	°F	°C
CBG	248	120
Delta-9 THC	314	157
CBD	320–356	160–180
CBDV	356	180
CBN	365	185
THCV	428	220
CBC	428	220

Terpenes	°F	°C
Humulene	252	122
Nerolidol	252	122
Beta-caryophyllene	266	130
Pinene	311	155
Myrcene	334	168
Limonene	349	176
Terpinolene	366	186
Linalool	388	198

Sourced from *Cannabis Drinks: Secrets to Crafting CBD and THC Beverages at Home*

A Note from Chef Haejin Chun
CANNABIS & KOREAN FLAVORS

Cannabis has been a significant part of my life for two decades. Representing my culture with intention, in both food and weed, is really important to me. Just like cannabis, Korean food is herbaceous. Creating pairings that are complementary and balanced is just as important as choosing any other ingredient or herb in your recipe. I love combining all the complexities and nuanced multitudes of weed with infused hot sauces, kimchis, broths, and dipping sauces. When pairing, I consider the terpene profile to be a flavor profile that you can use to build endless savory or sweet combinations—just like pairing rosemary and thyme with meat and poultry, or pairing basil with tomatoes and pasta. Whether you decide to pair cannabis alongside your meal or infuse it into a recipe, here are a few of my favorite strains that best complement the recipes in this book.

PINEAPPLE KUSH: I often pair this strain with Asian vinaigrettes or sauces for red meat, pork, or chicken. This strain is best known for its sour/sweet pineapple notes and minty undertones.

GARLIC BREATH: The name says it all—it smells and tastes like garlic! Super pungent, Garlic Breath enhances noodles, stews, chili oil, and hot sauce.

GELATO 41: Perfect for desserts and sweets! Think of a hint of citrus, berries, and cream.

WHITE TRUFFLE: Yes, you read that correctly: White Truffle! I love the savory, earthy, and umami notes of this strain, with a little bit of added funk. It's perfect for potatoes, pasta, popcorn butter, and more.

SUPER LEMON OG: This strain is very citrusy but with a subtle earthiness and the right amount of gas. It's great for almost any dish that could use a kiss of lemon or lime, but it pairs particularly well with seafood.

To further explore how to match cannabis with food and beverages, turn to page 32. Enjoy, and happy cooking!

DOSAGE GUIDE

No matter what cannabis products you're enjoying, it's crucial to be aware of how many phytocannabinoids you're consuming at any given time, especially when it comes to THC. With this in mind, it's imperative to understand the concept of dosing. For the unfamiliar, a dose refers to how much THC, CBD, or other active compounds are in your products. When purchasing cannabis from a legal market-licensed dispensary or delivery service, this information is required to be displayed on the packaging. We highly recommend that you source your products from a legitimate retailer so you have this information on hand (and ensure that you get safe, clean cannabis products to work with).

Cannabis impacts everyone differently, so no standard or universal dose works for everyone. A "perfect dose" completely depends on the person consuming the cannabis and is influenced by many factors, including body weight, metabolism, what you ate that day, how hydrated you are, and your body's natural chemical makeup. Tailoring your consumption to what specifically works best for your own body and your desired effects should be top of mind when you're first experimenting. Understanding your body's unique response and relationship to cannabis is crucial to building the right experience for you. The following dosage guide will help you get started, but when in doubt, always remember the golden rule: *Start low and go slow.*

AT-HOME DOSING 101

Understanding how to dose edibles and drinkables properly will ensure a pleasant experience when cooking with cannabis at home. Even the most experienced consumers know that it's very easy to go overboard without the proper guidelines, so it's vital to take the time to understand how to calculate the dose per serving based on the products you're using.

For the purposes of this book, the included recipes range between 5 and 10 milligrams of THC per serving. The target dose listed in each recipe can simply be a baseline for your infusions, but your final outcome will vary, depending on the flower or concentrate that you use. Based on your comfort level, you can adjust the potency up or down by following a few simple instructions (flip to page 27 to learn how to increase or decrease the potency of your infusions). If you're a newbie, we suggest staying between 1 and 5 milligrams per serving for THC.

For CBD, most people begin with 5 to 25 milligrams of CBD per edible or drinkable. This cannabinoid won't get you high like THC, so there's much more flexibility when experimenting. If you have access to cannabis products that contain both THC and CBD, these healing phytocannabinoids work together alongside the other natural compounds in cannabis to enhance each other's efficacy (refer back to page 10 to learn more about the *entourage effect*). If you're consuming both, modify the amount you are taking until you find a ratio that suits your personal preferences. The higher the amount of CBD to TCH means you'll be less high.

> *Tip!* To calculate the total amount of THC and CBD, you must first combine CBD + CBDA and THC + THCA percentages to estimate the potency of your infusions. This information should be listed on the packaging of the flower or concentrate when you purchase it or listed on the Certificate of Analysis (CoA), if available. To calculate, multiply the CBDA or THCA by a 0.877 conversion rate and add it to the amount of CBD and THC listed. If you don't see CBDA and THCA percentages listed on the packaging, then this conversion has already been done for you.

THE DOSAGE CALCULATION

When creating edibles and drinkables at home, use this step-by-step formula to calculate the dosage per serving (adapted from the book *The Ultimate Guide to CBD*). After you've done the math, always use measuring spoons, droppers, and cups to dose as accurately as possible. You can also access an online dosage calculator by visiting www.CannabisSpatula.com.

STEP 1: Convert THC and CBD percentages to determine milligrams per gram of dry flower (1 gram = 1,000 milligrams).
Example: Based on the values for Vanilla Frosting, 15% THC and 1% CBD
    0.15 x 1,000 mg/g = 150 mg THC per gram
    0.01 x 1,000 mg/g = 10 mg CBD per gram

STEP 2: Multiply the mg/g of THC and CBD from step 1 by the grams of flower called for in your recipe.
Example: For butter, a recipe calls for 3.5 grams of cannabis flower
    150 mg/g x 3.5 g = 525 mg THC
    10 mg/g x 3.5 g = 35 mg CBD

STEP 3: Convert your primary infusion ingredients (coconut oil, duck fat, olive oil, butter, high-proof alcohol, and so on) into grams.
Example: 1 cup butter = 227 grams
Here are some additional conversions, including olive oil, milk, water, and more:
    1 cup coconut oil/MCT oil = 216 grams
    1 cup Everclear = 216 grams
    1 cup olive oil = 219 grams
    1 cup water = 240 grams
    1 cup milk = 245 grams
    1 cup coconut milk = 250 grams

> *Tip!* **Keep in mind that you'll never be 100 percent accurate in determining the dosage. Many factors can vary the outcome, including heating methods, ingredients used, evaporation, and cannabinoid loss due decarboxylation and cooking. Use this formula as a rough estimate when preparing your infusions. Most times, the potency will be a little lower than this estimate due to cannabinoid loss during decarboxylation and loss of volume due to evaporation during the infusion process. To test it, we recommend sampling ⅛ to ¼ teaspoon (or whatever serving size you're comfortable with) to gauge the potency of your infusion before mixing it into a recipe and serving others. If you're using a concentrate, use this same formula, but sample a smaller amount; this type of infusion can be very potent. Safe and responsible dosing should always be top of mind.**

STEP 4: Calculate the number of servings remaining in your final yield. Divide your answer from step 3 by the number of grams per serving, indicated in the following chart.
Example: 227 g butter ÷ 14.18 g butter per tablespoon = About 16 tablespoons butter

Ingredient	Serving Size	Grams
Oil (olive, coconut, chili, and so on)	1 tablespoon	13.75
Butter	1 tablespoon	14.18
Milk	1 ounce	30.63
Simple syrup	1 ounce	28
Alcohol tincture	1 millimeter	0.789

STEP 5: Divide your THC and CBD amounts from step 2 by the number of servings in step 4 to calculate the THC and CBD per serving.
Example: Final calculation for butter
    525 mg ÷ 16 TB. = 32.8 mg THC per tablespoon, or 10.93 mg THC per teaspoon
    35 mg ÷ 16 TB. = About 2.2 mg CBD per tablespoon, or < 1 mg CBD per teaspoon

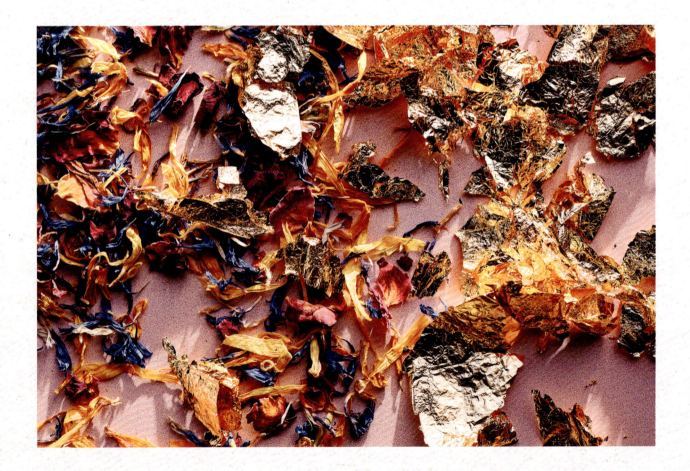

METHODS FOR INCREASING AND DECREASING THE POTENCY OF HOMEMADE INFUSIONS

Because cannabis is a personalized plant and not "one size fits all," it's important to know the methods for increasing or decreasing the potency of homemade infusions, to ensure that you're working with a dosage that you're comfortable with. The recipes included in this book range between 5 and 10 milligrams THC, but you can easily customize your own dose by following these tips to best accommodate your needs. Whatever method you choose, be sure to calculate the dosage to estimate the updated potency.

Increasing the Potency

- **USE LESS LIQUID TO INCREASE THE POTENCY.** To increase the potency, you can concentrate your infusions by using less liquid during the heating process. Just keep in mind that this strategy will also concentrate any cannabis flavors, so your infusions might taste more green/dank.

- **CHOOSE THC-RICH STRAINS.** To create the most potent infusions, pay close attention to how much THC is in the product you're working with, and choose something that's THC-rich. Anything 20 percent THC or higher will yield a stronger homemade infusion. Common THC-rich strains: Gelato, OG Kush, Kush Mints, GMO Cookies, Trainwreck

- **USE PROFESSIONALLY MADE HIGH-POTENCY PRODUCTS.** If you're someone who requires more than 100 milligrams per serving, it's recommended that you incorporate your favorite store-bought high-potency products into your recipes, such as a tincture or RSO. This will allow you to precisely dose based on your needs. Just be sure to take extra precautions when working with high levels of THC, and consume in a safe, comfortable space.

Decreasing the Potency

- **DILUTE YOUR INFUSION.** To decrease the potency, one of the simplest strategies is to dilute the infusion using additional noninfused oil, butter, or other pantry item ingredient you're infusing. Simply combine your desired amount with the cannabis-infused version, and mix well. If you're diluting a fat-based infusion that solidifies (such as butter or coconut oil), you can combine over low heat and then cool to solidify again before serving. You can dilute as much as you'd like in order to reach your desired dosage range.

- **CHOOSE CBD-RICH STRAINS AND PRODUCTS.** If you're looking to avoid high amounts of THC, we recommend seeking out CBD-rich strains and products to combine into your infusions. Some of the most common high CBD/low THC ratios include 20:1 (pronounced "twenty to one"), 18:1, 8:1, 4:1, 3:1, and 1:1 for a more balanced experience. If you'd rather avoid THC altogether, hemp-derived broad-spectrum items and CBD isolates are other options. Just keep in mind that you'll be missing out on the entourage effect (page 10) and the combined healing elements of cannabis.
Common CBD-rich strains: ACDC, Cannatonic, Charlotte's Web, Harlequin, Harle-Tsu

HOW TO SAFELY SERVE INFUSED FOODS & BEVERAGES

One of the joys of cooking with cannabis is sharing infused treats with family and friends. When offering cannabis-infused foods and beverages to others, the following are a few precautions and recommendations to keep in mind.

PRECAUTIONS & RECOMMENDATIONS FROM THE PROS

ALWAYS ASK QUESTIONS! No matter what the occasion is, communication is key when serving others. If you're planning to offer infused food or drinks to a group, always get a verbal confirmation from your guests on their comfort level with cannabis. Not everyone wants to consume THC (or CBD), so make communication a priority before, during, and after the event to ensure a pleasurable experience. Ask any and all questions to verify your guests' comfort levels.

EDUCATE YOUR GUESTS ON THE GOLDEN RULE: *Start low, go slow.* When serving cannabis-infused items to guests, make sure that they're aware of the Golden Rule and that they know to be patient when consuming edibles and drinkables. It can take anywhere from 30 minutes to 2 hours for full effects to set in, so communicate this to your guests to ensure that they don't overdo it.

SAMPLE INFUSIONS BEFORE SERVING THEM TO OTHERS. As previously discussed, you should always sample your infusions before combining them into a recipe and serving to others. We recommend sampling a day or two prior to hosting the event so you have time to adjust the potency (and to avoid being too high on event day).

LABEL EVERYTHING. When creating infused items, always add labels and clearly mark whether the item contains cannabis. This is incredibly important, especially if you share a refrigerator, freezer, or pantry space with other people. Be sure your infused items are stored safely and away from places where children can access them. You should also clearly label all cannabis food and beverage items that are served at events. If you're tray-passing these items, have your servers further communicate the dosage per serving to your guests, keeping communication top of mind.

IF YOU'RE SERVING MULTIPLE INFUSED ITEMS, STICK TO A LOW DOSE PER COURSE OR PER APPETIZER. By offering a lower dose, your guests will be able to enjoy the full meal without getting too high and taste multiple appetizers without worry. For passed appetizers, dosing between 1 and 2 milligrams per serving is recommended (and remember, always communicate with your guests that the food is infused!). For a coursed meal, dosing the food is more strategic and depends on what type of experience you're looking to create. Some chefs prefer serving multiple courses at 1 to 2 milligrams of THC per course; others dose at higher levels or incorporate minor cannabinoids throughout the meal. Depending on who you're serving the infused meal to, know your audience and their comfort levels.

ALWAYS HAVE CBD AVAILABLE, IN CASE SOMEONE GETS TOO HIGH. If you're serving cannabis products to others, have some high-quality CBD on hand in case someone gets too high. CBD won't make you "unhigh," but it can counteract some of the negative side effects of consuming too much THC, such as anxiety and paranoia. When consuming both phytocannabinoids together, CBD weakens THC's ability to bind with CB1 receptors, thus softening THC's effects. This is why you feel more balanced when consuming products that contain *both* CBD and THC versus a product that contains only THC.

BE SURE TO HAVE PLENTY OF DRINKING WATER AVAILABLE. Dehydration can quickly escalate into a bad experience. Keeping your guests hydrated is one of the most important things you can do as a responsible event host. When people get high, they get thirsty, so be sure to have fresh water available at all times.

ADVICE FOR SERVING CANNABIS AND ALCOHOL: If you're planning to serve both cannabis and alcohol, take precautions and do so carefully. When enjoying these powerful substances together, it's all about moderation. Combining the two can be quite enjoyable, but educate your guests so that they're aware of the potential negative side effects of getting dizzy and sick if they consume too much of either. *Take it slow.* If you're serving THC-infused cocktails that contain alcohol, stay below 10 milligrams of THC per drink, or between 1 and 2.5 milligrams of THC for beginners. For more tips on how best to combine cannabis and alcohol into a cocktail, flip to page 131.

Cannabis Chef's Checklist

Now that you've mastered the most important cannabis cooking essentials, here's a final checklist to review before you start cooking. To set yourself up for success, follow these four tips:

- ☐ **KEEP YOUR WORK AREA CLEAN AND ORGANIZED.** In general, timing is important when baking and cooking. Make sure you have everything you need before you start.

- ☐ **CHECK YOUR CANNABIS.** Make sure your flower is fresh and clean before incorporating it into an infusion. Look and smell for mold. If your flower smells off, is damp but not sticky, or has turned a brownish color, do not use it! Bad weed will ruin your infusions.

- ☐ **PREP YOUR OVEN, AND ALWAYS DOUBLE-CHECK THE HEAT.** Before preheating, place your rack in the middle of the oven for an even temperature. After preheating, if you have an oven that heats via a dial (in 25° increments), be sure to use a thermometer to double-check the temperature. Remember, every degree counts when cooking with cannabis!

- ☐ **WEAR GLOVES.** Touching cannabis won't make you feel high, but the compounds can still be absorbed through the skin. Most people are fine when smoking or eating weed, but touching the plant or having the oils on your skin can cause irritation or a small allergic reaction. For this reason, be sure to wear gloves when cooking with herbal products.

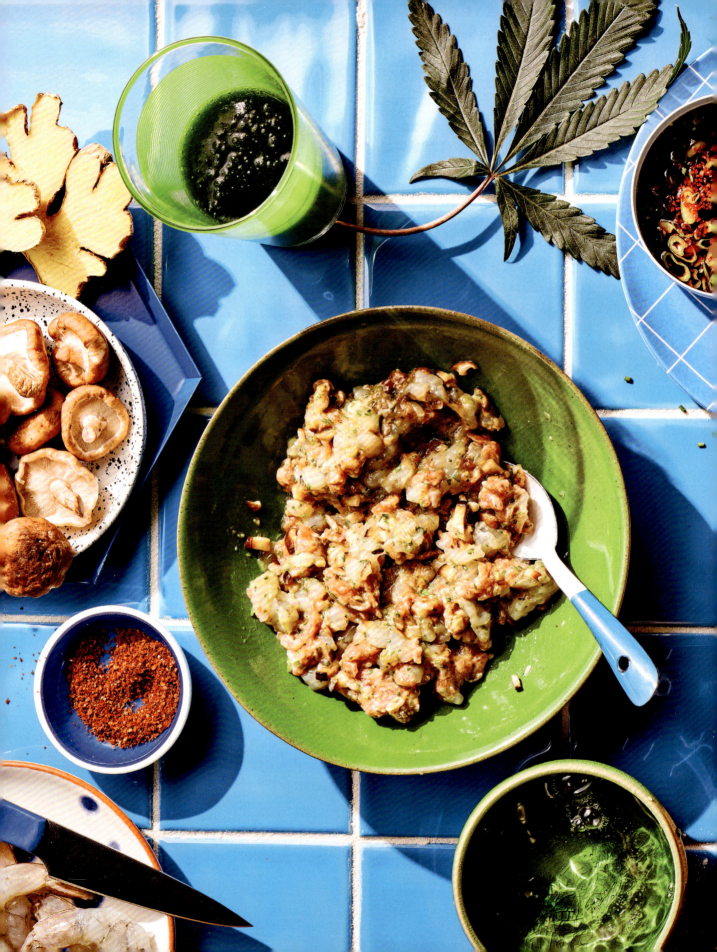

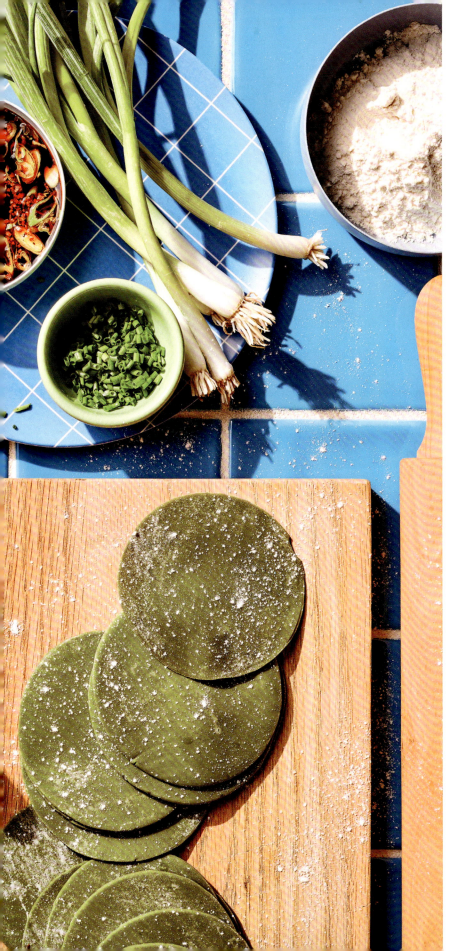

THE ART OF COOKING WITH CANNABIS

CHAPTER 2

Although it is still a somewhat untapped and uncommon culinary item, cannabis is making its way into cuisines across the globe. Both at-home cooks and professional chefs are pushing new boundaries of the culinary cannabis world, creating innovative cannabis-infused meals that go beyond your typical pot brownie.

Cannabis is both an art and a science. This section will help you discover how to choose the best cannabis ingredients, learn tips for pairing cannabis with your meal, explore must-have ingredients, plus master the art of creating cannabis infusions. Ready to elevate your cooking with cannabis? Let's dig in!

COMBINING CANNABIS WITH FOOD

Similar to cooking with other fresh herbs, creating quality infusions begins with quality ingredients. It's important to source cannabis from the legal market at a licensed dispensary or delivery service that is lab tested and accompanied by a Certificate of Analysis (CoA), to ensure that the material you're working with is clean. When you feel confident about the products you've selected, you can start combining cannabis with food and beverages. First, here's a guide to the most common cannabis ingredients.

CHOOSE YOUR CANNABIS INGREDIENT

If you're new to cannabis and are unsure of what type of product to use when baking and cooking, pay close attention to this section! Choosing the right cannabis products based on your personal needs is the first essential step in preparing infused recipes. Whether you're curious to learn more about cannabis flower or you want to experiment with more potent concentrates, this section has something for everyone. If you're a cannabis pro and you know your products well, feel free to jump ahead to page 40 to start preparing the infusions.

Cannabis Flower

Whether you're inhaling or infusing into a recipe, enjoying cannabis flower is one of the most tried-and-true ways to consume cannabis. This magical herb is available in thousands of cultivars, each displaying a vast array of phytocannabinoids, terpenes, and effects. If you're just beginning your cannabis journey, the number of strains available can seem overwhelming, which is why it's incredibly important to know how to select the best cannabis flower for your particular needs. Here are some key points to keep in mind:

YOUR NOSE KNOWS: One of the best ways to determine what strain is right for you is to smell the actual cannabis buds to see what aromas resonate with you. Whatever smells best is often an indication of what cannabis terpene profile your body is craving. As we say in the cannabis industry, your nose knows! However, based on where you're located, smelling cannabis or hemp flower before you purchase it might not be possible, due to federal or state regulations. In these circumstances, it's best to research the specific effect you're trying to achieve and then consult with a budtender or cannabis concierge to help you choose the best products. We also recommend keeping a strain journal so you can keep track of what works best for you.

INDICA VS. SATIVA: When choosing a cannabis product, consumers are often limited to selecting an indica or sativa. Although this terminology is much more relevant to cultivators than to consumers, it has been the primary way products have been marketed, based on "predictable" effects. To clarify, this is not a very accurate way to determine how cannabis will make you feel. As it turns out, the majority of cannabis flower that's available is a hybrid of the two. To truly determine how a strain will make you feel, it's best to pay attention to the total combination of phytocannabinoids and terpenes.

SUN-GROWN VS. INDOOR CANNABIS: Whether you are team sun-grown or team indoor, both growing methods are continually up for debate on what produces superior cannabis. In our opinion, nothing is better than celebrating the bounty of what Mother Nature has gifted us and embracing sun-grown cannabis, especially when cooking or mixing up drinks.

From a chef and mixologist's point of view, you can smell and taste the difference between sun-grown and indoor cannabis, which directly translates to your recipes if you prepare your infusions correctly. There's a robust freshness to sun-grown flower that can be produced only by living soil, the alchemy of a direct kiss from the sun, and a growing region's sense of place (otherwise known as *terroir*). As with any other high-quality ingredients at their prime, we are strong proponents of farm-to-table cooking. Cannabis is no different.

To put this into perspective, think of a sun-grown tomato versus a tomato that has been grown indoors. The tomato will properly grow only by assimilating the conditions of an outdoor garden, with eight hours of sunlight per day at a temperature of around 70°F (21°C) or higher. Although indoor growing offers some advantage due to this hypercontrolled environment, synthetically replicating these conditions is not only unsustainable, but also incredibly expensive. Indoor plants miss out on the full spectrum of natural sunlight and the abundant benefits of living soil (soil that contains microbial life, including fungi, bacteria, protozoa, and many other beneficial organisms), one of the key ingredients to growing the best cannabis.

Farmers who produce sun-grown cannabis also holistically and dynamically tend to the land. They believe in regenerative farming, incorporating permaculture and organic/biodynamic farming practices to rebuild soil and organic matter to preserve the land for future generations. These thoughtful practices contribute to world-class cannabis, which is why the farms in the Emerald Triangle (Humboldt, Mendocino, and Trinity counties in California) produce some of the best cannabis in the world. All of these methods make a difference that you can smell and taste. When working with cannabis as an ingredient, choose sun-grown if you have the option.

If you live in a region that does not offer sun-grown cannabis, look for sustainable flower that's lab tested and clean certified. We also recommend supporting brands that you love and that align with your values.

A Note from Jamie Evans, The Herb Somm
HOW TO MATCH FLOWER WITH FLAVORS

With so many aromatic and flavorful properties of cannabis, it's easy to pair your favorite strains with food, beverages, and other ingredients. Just as a sommelier matches wine to a meal, you can use a similar approach to create the best cannabis pairings. To do so properly, it's important to be familiar with the most common terpene profiles (flip to page 19 for an overview) and learn how to recognize their unique characteristics in cannabis. Think of this practice as sensory training, as you train your nose and palate to pick out different nuances, just as in wine tasting. Here's a fun exercise to try at home:

CANNABIS SENSORY TRAINING 101: When learning how to pair flower with other ingredients, the first step is evaluating the cannabis on its own. While at home, leave the cannabis in its jar or transfer it to a wine glass to best evaluate the aromas. Place your nose just above the top of the jar or inside the wine glass, and briefly breathe in several times (like you're emulating a bunny). Repeat this smelling exercise a few times to best evaluate all the layers of aromas the cannabis strain presents (almost like you're evaluating wine!). If you're unable to pick up on the notes at first, break up some of the flower using your fingers to release a burst of terpenes. Take notes of everything you're discovering. Next, it's time to taste the flower. To best evaluate the true flavors of the terpene profile, taking a "dry pull" from a joint or using a dry flower vaporizer is recommended. Both of these techniques avoid combustion (lighting the cannabis with a flame), to better preserve these precious compounds so you can taste them. If you're unfamiliar with the dry pull, place a joint to your lips and inhale (without lighting the joint). You'll quickly be able to taste the terpene profile of the cannabis strain you're enjoying without inhaling smoke (this technique will not get you high). When you're done evaluating the terpene profile, feel free to light up the joint and enjoy.

While you're evaluating the flower, some of the most common aromas and flavors to look for include citrus fruits (lemon, lime, grapefruit, tangerine), earthy notes (mushroom, forest floor, fresh soil), floral notes (lavender, citrus blossom, roses), baking spices (cinnamon, nutmeg, black pepper), and fresh herbs (rosemary, dill, mint), among other herbal, floral, fruit, and spice notes. If you're able to recognize some of these smells and tastes in cannabis, you've successfully identified terpenes. Now it's time to create the pairing.

Whether you decide to complement or contrast with the ingredients in your dish or cocktail, the best part of matching cannabis flower with flavors is to be creative. Don't be afraid to experiment to see what works best with each menu and occasion. Trying to mask the flavors of cannabis when cooking or making drinks will not produce the greatest outcome. Instead, use terpene-rich ingredients to amplify the natural aromas and flavors of the herbal products you're working with to yield the most delicious combinations.

CONCENTRATES

Concentrates are processed, highly potent, condensed cannabis products that separate or extract all the cannabinoids from excess plant matter into a concentrated mass, leaving you with a pure-form, full-flavor product that packs a punch! Simply put, they are the concentrated form of cannabis, containing a much higher level of cannabinoids and terpenes than other types of products. Most flower averages at about 15 to 25 percent THC; concentrates contain as much as 50 to 90 percent THC. Because of this, a stigma persists, even among seasoned consumers, that concentrates can be intimidating. However, when you learn more about this topic and how to safely work with concentrates, you will find many perks to using this form of cannabis.

If you're dabbing or smoking concentrates, you can achieve a maximum high for a minimum amount of smoke/intake. Although there isn't enough research to make a final conclusion, some experts even say that concentrates might be better for your lungs. There's also less smoke because you're not burning plant matter, so smoking concentrates is less odorous than consuming flower.

As an ingredient in a recipe, concentrates retain the highest amount of flavor due to the preservation of terpenes during the extraction process. Because the plant matter has already been removed, you can also skip the straining/filtering process, which is normally required when infusing with whole cannabis flower.

No matter which concentrate you choose, using these products is one of the easiest methods of cooking with cannabis because it involves fewer steps and less mess. Additionally, concentrates have complex, intense flavors, which are considered the liquid gold form of cannabis. That makes working with concentrates a chef's dream because they're such a pure, decadent form of cannabis.

The Best Concentrates to Cook With

Solventless concentrates are cannabis extracts made without the use of chemical solvents such as butane or CO_2. By using solventless cannabis, you can avoid potentially harmful additives in your food or beverages. If you're looking to incorporate solventless concentrates into your cooking, here are some of the best types to work with (continue reading for other concentrates you should avoid, page 36):

- **KIEF:** Dried but sticky trichome crystals that naturally fall off the plant. They can be accumulated by sifting the plant through a screen or fine-mesh sieve. Kief is a great product to use when you don't want to add too much liquid to your infusion (for example, when using honey).

- **ICE WATER HASH/BUBBLE HASH:** Made by rigorously agitating cannabis flower with ice and water. This process shakes off the trichomes and separates the resin/oil from the plant matter. Ice water hash is great for lower-temp infusions, such as butter infusions.

- **LIVE ROSIN:** A type of hash. Not to be confused with live resin, which is not solventless. *Live* refers to the use of fresh-frozen flower, which is cultivated at its peak and then immediately frozen (instead of being dried or cured) to preserve the freshness of the plant (think of the difference between dried basil and freshly frozen basil). Heated plates are then used to slowly press out the oils. Live rosin is the perfect match for higher-temperature oils such as coconut oil, avocado oil, and bacon fat.

> *Tip!* These solventless concentrates can all be used interchangeably, based on what you have access to; there's no wrong answer, although temperature control is important (turn to page 22).

Concentrates to Avoid

When cooking with cannabis, we recommend staying away from the following concentrates because it's easier for manufacturers to hide fillers that can impact your health. Avoid using the following: butane/solvents, distillates, and diamonds.

Isolates

If you're seeking isolated phytocannabinoids, meaning a single cannabinoid without any other compounds present, cooking or baking with an isolate is another method for infusing recipes. Most commonly available as CBD in a powdered form, isolates can be easily incorporated into butter, oil, and other heated infusions, as well as blended into food and drinks. If you're planning to use an isolate, pay attention to the milligrams per serving; some products can reach high dosages quickly. However, be aware that you're missing out on the entourage effect (refer to page 10) and the combined healing elements of cannabis, which might not be as effective as with some of the other full-spectrum options available, including flower, concentrates, and tinctures.

Tinctures

Whether you're purchasing a commercially made product or creating one at home, using a tincture to infuse a recipe is a fantastic way to incorporate cannabis into a number of your favorite foods and beverages. If you're working with a commercially made tincture, you'll most often find oil-based options available that seamlessly combine into baking recipes. Commercially made tinctures also allow for precise dosing because you can easily titrate the milligrams per dose up or down until you find your perfect ratio. Just be sure you're using an *unflavored* tincture; some products are heavily infused with botanicals and other flavors, which can impact the outcome of your recipe.

In this book, you also discover how to create your own tinctures at home using alcohol as the solvent. Learning the steps to create this type of tincture is one of the best ways to infuse beverages and other liquid-based recipes. Just keep in mind that homemade tinctures will never yield a precise dose, so always be sure to calculate the estimated dosage, depending on what cannabis material you're working with. Flip to page 58 for two methods of creating an alcohol-based tincture at home.

Commercially Made Gourmet Cannabis Products

If making an infusion seems totally out of your comfort zone, don't fret! Commercially made gourmet cannabis products will jumpstart your baking game in no time. Depending on what's available in your state or country, various cannabis-infused pantry items can be used to easily infuse food and beverages. Some of the most popular items include professionally made cannabis-infused olive oil, honey, sugar, chili oil, and sweet, savory, or spicy sauces. Not only are these products delicious, but they're also incredibly easy to use and offer precise dosing, thanks to stringent lab testing requirements. Just be sure to use measuring spoons or cups for the most accurate measurements. Flip to page 169 for a listing of our favorite gourmet cannabis products out at the time of writing this book.

BUILDING YOUR CANNABIS PANTRY

Now that you're familiar with some of the most common cannabis ingredients to cook with, it's time to build your cannabis pantry. Whether you choose to make infusions using cannabis flower, concentrates, or something else, follow these essential tips to ensure that you're choosing the best products possible.

Six Tips for Choosing the Best Products

1. **DO YOUR OWN RESEARCH.** When it comes to sourcing cannabis products, do your own research to determine what type of product will work best for your needs. Whether you're looking for something to help with sleep or reduce anxiety, learn as much information as you can on your own; then save any remaining questions for an expert budtender at a licensed dispensary. With basic knowledge, you'll be better equipped to get the best bang for your buck, and the budtender won't be able to steer you blindly to promotional products. Keep in mind that not everything on the internet is factual, so be sure you're sourcing your information from multiple, reputable sources and comparing your findings. Flip to page 169 for a listing of some of the most trusted educational resources.

2. **ALWAYS LOOK AT PACKAGING DATES TO DETERMINE FRESHNESS.** Like anything with a shelf life, it's incredibly important to look at packaging and expiration dates to best gauge freshness. If it was harvested and packaged recently, the cannabis should present exuberant terpene notes, with aromas bursting out of the jar. If the packaging dates are old, chances are good that the volatile terpenes have diminished and the phytocannabinoids have oxidized, which is not ideal. If you're sourcing from a licensed retailer, this information is required to be listed on the packaging, so look at dates before you buy!

3. **MAKE SURE PRODUCTS ARE CLEAN AND LAB TESTED.** We previously touched on this topic in Chapter 1, but always source clean, lab-tested products from a reliable resource anytime you're enjoying cannabis. If you source a cannabis product that has not been tested, there's a chance that it could contain dangerous pesticides and heavy metals that might impact your health. A lower price tag on these items might tempt you, but be your own advocate and protect your health by staying away from these products. Always choose lab-tested items that come with a legitimate Certificate of Analysis (CoA).

4. **LOOK FOR ARTISANAL INSTEAD OF MASS-PRODUCED PRODUCTS.** We are forever supporters of the concept of *quality* over *quantity*. When sourcing cannabis products, the best and most flavorful items almost always come from artisanal producers who are masters of their craft and genuinely care about what they are producing. You can smell, taste, and feel the intention that has gone into creating these small-batch products, which directly transfers into your recipes.

5. **HIGH THC CONTENT DOESN'T ALWAYS MEAN IT'S A BETTER PRODUCT.** When purchasing cannabis, THC content is often the first thing people look for to determine whether it's a good product. THC percentages help you gauge potency, but they can't tell you what kind of effect you're going to experience. This just isn't the best way to evaluate the overall efficacy of cannabis or how it will interact with your body. Instead of looking at just one piece of the puzzle (THC), consider the full spectrum of phytocannabinoids and terpenes that are in the product to best meet your personal needs.

6. **SUPPORT THE BRANDS YOU BELIEVE IN.** Always support the brands you believe in and purchase items from companies that align with your values. We are proponents of women-owned and equity brands, as well as artisanal sun-grown cannabis farms. Flip to page 169 for a listing of some of our favorite producers and products.

SHOPPING GUIDE CHECKLISTS

Before you put on that apron, look over our must-have checklists to assist with sourcing equipment and ingredients to be used throughout this book. Be sure to check your kitchen, pantry, spice cabinet, and refrigerator to see what you already have on hand before you head to the store. If you don't have all these items, no problem! You can still prepare the recipes with a little creative improv. For example, if you don't own cheesecloth to strain the solids from your infusion, you can easily swap for a single-ply paper towel sheet lined in a strainer, which will catch the small particles when you're filtering your infusions. This is just one example of how you can work with what you have. Be sure to reference the notes section found in each recipe for other helpful tips and tricks. Here's *almost* everything you'll need:

Essential Equipment

As you work your way through the food and drink recipes throughout this book, here's a master checklist of equipment to have on hand.

FOOD EQUIPMENT

- [ ] Chef's knife
- [ ] Different sizes of deli containers for prep
- [ ] Digital scale
- [ ] Foil
- [ ] Food-grade disposable gloves
- [ ] Freezer-grade plastic zip bags
- [ ] Lots of clean towels
- [ ] Measuring cups
- [ ] Measuring spoons
- [ ] Microplane
- [ ] Mixer
- [ ] Mixing bowls
- [ ] Parchment paper
- [ ] Paring knife
- [ ] Pots and pans
- [ ] Separate cutting boards for meat and produce
- [ ] Sheet trays
- [ ] Strainer
- [ ] Whisk

DRINK EQUIPMENT

- [ ] Amber glass bottles with dropper caps
- [ ] Bar spoon
- [ ] Blender or food processor
- [ ] Candy or instant-read thermometer
- [ ] Cheesecloth
- [ ] Citrus press
- [ ] Digital scale
- [ ] Double jigger
- [ ] Fine-mesh strainer
- [ ] Funnel
- [ ] Glass syrup bottle with stainless steel pourer
- [ ] Hawthorne strainer
- [ ] Mason jars of varying sizes
- [ ] Measuring glass (1 to 5 ounces)
- [ ] Mixing glass
- [ ] Muddler
- [ ] Oven mitt
- [ ] Peeler
- [ ] Saucepans of varying sizes
- [ ] Shaker tin
- [ ] Sous vide precision cooker
- [ ] Spice grinder
- [ ] Vacuum sealer
- [ ] Vacuum seal bags
- [ ] Whisk

Must-Have Ingredients to Have on Hand

Every recipe calls for several different types of ingredients. Here's a list of some of the most important items to have on hand (and used in multiple recipes). You can find most of these items at your local supermarket, but you might need to source some items online or at a specialty grocery store.

FOOD INGREDIENTS

- ☐ All-purpose flour
- ☐ Black pepper
- ☐ Black sesame
- ☐ Brown sugar
- ☐ Butter
- ☐ Chives
- ☐ Coconut cream
- ☐ Fish sauce
- ☐ Garlic
- ☐ Ginger
- ☐ Gochujang
- ☐ Korean chili flakes
- ☐ Mirin
- ☐ Rice wine vinegar
- ☐ Sesame oil
- ☐ Soy sauce
- ☐ Star anise
- ☐ White miso (no dashi)
- ☐ White sugar

DRINK INGREDIENTS

- ☐ Butter
- ☐ Bittering agents (cinchona bark, horehound)
- ☐ Citrus fruits (blood oranges, lemons, limes, grapefruits)
- ☐ Chocolate
- ☐ Club soda or sparkling water
- ☐ Coconut milk
- ☐ Cream of coconut
- ☐ Dairy or nondairy milk (whole milk, coconut, soymilk milk)
- ☐ Food-grade vegetable glycerin
- ☐ Fresh cannabis leaves (the best place to source cannabis leaves is to grow your own plants!)
- ☐ Fresh fruits (pineapple, peaches, raspberries, watermelon)
- ☐ Fresh juices (pineapple, passion fruit, tomato)
- ☐ Fresh and dried herbs (mint, shiso)
- ☐ Ginger
- ☐ High-proof grain alcohol (clear and unflavored, beginning at 120 proof)
- ☐ Honey (or other natural sweeteners, such as agave nectar)
- ☐ Hot peppers (serrano or jalapeño)
- ☐ Peanut butter chips
- ☐ Salts and seasonings (margarita salt, chili pepper/lime salt)
- ☐ Spices (cinnamon, turmeric, nutmeg, cardamom)
- ☐ Spirits (bourbon, tequila, rum, vodka, gin)
- ☐ Sugar (both brown and granulated)
- ☐ Vanilla extract

> *Tip!* Make sure all the glass you use during your infusions is tempered glass, meaning it's been treated to withstand high temperatures without cracking or breaking. Don't let that hard work and high-quality product go to waste because your glass explodes and your infused oil spills all over the counter and floor. We learned this the hard way (oops!).

CREATING INFUSIONS 101

Welcome to the infusions section! Now that you have a solid understanding of how to work with cannabis as an ingredient, it's time to start cooking. As you've learned (page 32), the best way to incorporate cannabis into food and beverages is to create an infusion by combining cannabis with an alcohol- or fat-based solution to extract phytocannabinoids, terpenes, and other healing compounds. To do this successfully at home, here's an overview of the best extraction ingredients to use, as well as the most popular methods for preparing infusions. If you're already familiar with these concepts, flip to page 72 for the food infusion recipes or page 126 for the drink infusion recipes.

Extraction Ingredients

Whether you're working with an oil, a butter, or alcohol, these everyday extraction ingredients (also known as *solvents*) will act as your most favored and reliable pantry items to create cannabis infusions at home. Fat-based solutions are especially helpful when baking and cooking. Luckily, phytocannabinoids such as THC and CBD are naturally drawn to fats, making them lipophilic, or fat-soluble compounds. This is why so many cannabis products are currently made with oil and why cannabis combines so well with butter!

These compounds can also be extracted using an alcohol such as bourbon or a high-proof grain alcohol, which is the most suitable way to combine cannabis-infused ingredients into a beverage or cocktail. Depending on what extraction ingredient you're using, the following are important things to keep in mind before mixing with cannabis.

Oil

When creating oil infusions at home, feel free to use whatever oil you'd like. In this book, you learn how to infuse olive oil, coconut oil, sesame oil, avocado oil, and chili oil. Although the method for infusing remains consistent, pay close attention to the boiling point of each type of oil, and stay far below this number to best preserve phytocannabinoids, terpenes, and the overall quality of the oil you're working with. Depending on the oil's flavor, you can also pair the notes of the oil with a complementing cannabis strain to create an out-of-this-world delicious and unique infusion! For the oil infusions, flip to page 44.

Butter

Cannabis-infused butter is the most common baking ingredient to make because it effortlessly combines into just about any baking recipe that calls for traditional butter. For the best extraction, source a high-fat butter (such as European butter, with a minimum of 82 percent fat) to bind with cannabis compounds when heated together. In general, we also recommend using *unsalted* butter for your infusions to monitor how much salt is going into the final recipe. Unlike other oils, butter is more delicate and begins changing in texture and flavor to varying degrees, which can affect the depth and flavor of your dish. Butter begins to separate at 160°F (71°C) and starts to brown at 250°F (121°C), which are pretty low temperatures to be aware of. Turn to page 48 for a butter infusion recipe.

Alcohol

When using alcohol to extract cannabis compounds, it's vital to pay close attention to your extraction method, particularly if heat is involved. Alcohol is extremely flammable, especially with high-proof alcohol, so it's best to either stick with a nonheated option for creating the infusion, such as the mason jar method (see page 59), or use a sous vide to heat the infusion in a warm bath at low temperatures for a quicker turnaround time. If you decide to heat alcohol, never use a gas stove, and closely watch cooking temperatures. Heat the infusion well below 170°F (77°C) because alcohol flames at this point. In this book, you learn how to craft several different types of alcohol infusions, including tinctures and bitters. Jump to page 56 for the infusion recipes and page 29 for other tips and precautions when mixing cannabis with alcohol.

Other Considerations

Every now and then, you come across an infusion that does not traditionally contain an alcohol- or fat-based solution, such as simple syrup (typically made from water and a sugar base). In these situations, you can get creative and add some secret ingredients to assist with the extraction process. One of these secret ingredients is food-grade glycerin. When creating a simple syrup, add 1 to 2 tablespoon of vegetable glycerin during the heating process; it will bind with phytocannabinoids, terpenes, and other cannabis compounds.

When cooking or baking, keep a close eye on temperatures. Many ovens and stovetops have variable heat, so temperature control is incredibly important and will lead to a successful infusion. To best keep track of the heat, we recommend having an instant-read thermometer on hand for all the infusions included in this book. This tool is especially useful when heating any type of oil because temperatures can increase rapidly.

When you have your infusions ready, think about how and when you're going to infuse your dish. Will it be in the sauce or the marinade? Remember, cooking with high heat can burn off all those precious terpenes and phytocannabinoids you worked so hard to preserve. It's best to think ahead and choose the part of the dish with the least heat and resistance. For example, if you're making a grilled chicken salad, using infused oil or butter on the chicken before grilling is less optimal than infusing the salad dressing, which is the final step with *no heat*. Doing this ensures the preservation of your infusion in its full glory and is also the most accurate way to know that your dosage is correct.

METHODS FOR PREPARING INFUSIONS

If you've been researching how to cook with cannabis at home, you've most likely come across the many ways to prepare an infusion. Depending on what equipment you have on hand, you can choose from several approaches to working with the plant, as long as you have the essential ingredients (in other words, your choice of cannabis and the extraction ingredient). Before we reach the recipes, here's an overview of the most common methods used and some of the methods highlighted throughout this book.

The Stovetop Method

As the most common method for creating a heated infusion at home, the stovetop method is a reliable way to incorporate cannabis into oil, butter, simple syrup, and more. Using kitchen items you most likely already own, including a stove, saucepan, thermometer, and rubber spatula, you can easily prepare a number of infused recipes, as long as you keep a close eye on cooking temperatures and stir your infusion while it's cooking to evenly extract phytocannabinoids and terpenes. This method is approachable for both beginners and experts, but it can be time consuming because you have to monitor your infusion during the heating process (which, at times, can be several hours). For best results, stay between 160°F and 180°F (71°C and 82°C) when heating on the stovetop, and be careful not to exceed 200°F (93°C). Flip to page 44 for a recipe using the stovetop method.

Sous Vide

As discussed in Chapter 1, using a sous vide is a fantastic way to decarboxylate cannabis and prepare an infusion with minimal monitoring and odor. This portable cooking device allows for consistent heating at lower temperatures in a warm bath, preserving the integrity of your ingredients. If you're planning to use this method, be sure to have a vacuum sealer/vacuum seal zip bags (or tempered glass jars) on hand to heat the ingredients in. Simply set the sous vide to the recommended temperature in a water bath. After preheating the water, add your zip bag pouch or tempered glass jar to the bath and heat as directed. As a reminder, if you're working with alcohol, using a sous vide to heat the infusion is by far the safest method. Never heat alcohol over an open flame! Turn to page 44 for a recipe using the sous vide method.

Infusion Device

This method is for people who prefer to create infusions at the click of a button! If you have the resources to purchase an infusion device, this easy-to-use machine does all the hard work for you. You simply add your ingredients to the device, set the temperature and cooking time, and then press Go! Currently, many different brands of devices are available, with multiple settings and capabilities, making heating cannabis an easier task. Flip to page 169 for a listing of the infusion devices that are available at the time of writing this book.

Slow Cooker

If you have a slow cooker at home, guess what? You can use it to make cannabis infusions! This method is useful for cooking oil or butter at *low temperatures* and *slowly*. The only downside is, most slow cookers have limited temperature options, so dialing in a precise temperature isn't feasible. If you're planning to use this method, set the slow cooker on the lowest temperature setting, and then add the decarboxylated cannabis and your extraction ingredient. Cover the slow cooker, and heat as directed. Just be sure to use a thermometer to test the temperature so that you have an accurate read and can adjust accordingly.

The "Old-School" Mason Jar Method

When you're creating an alcohol infusion, one of the easiest ways to extract compounds is to combine decarboxylated cannabis with high-proof grain alcohol in a mason jar and store it in a cool, dark place, shaking the infusion from time to time (no heat required!). This "old-school" method of extraction has been used for centuries. Even Ancient Egyptians soaked herbs in alcohol to create healing tinctures and potions. If you're planning to make an alcohol-based infusion and you don't own a sous vide, using a mason jar will yield the same results. However, when using the mason jar method, the infusion process takes *a lot longer* (sometimes more than a week versus a couple hours using the sous vide). It's an incredibly common and easy method that requires very little equipment—you just have to be patient!

Infusion Recipes

Now that you have a thorough understanding of the cannabis cooking essentials and the various ways to create infusions, it's time to put your skills to the test! This section includes both food and drink infusion recipes that are used throughout this book. For food, you learn how to create various infused oils (olive oil, coconut oil, sesame oil, avocado oil, and chili oil), butter, honey, sugar, and infused saturated fat. In the beverage section, you'll master the art of creating cannabis-infused bitters, tinctures, simple syrup, coconut milk, fruit syrup, and fat-washed infusions. When you've assembled these important cannabis-infused pantry items, you can pretty much enhance just about any recipe.

> *Tip!* In this chapter, we infused the recipes using cannabis flower that measured at a total of 15 to 20 percent THC and 0 to 1 percent CBD before decarboxylation. Keep in mind, the target dosages included in each recipe can be used as a baseline for your infusions, but depending on the flower, concentrate, or other cannabis product you're using, your final outcome will vary. Always calculate the estimated milligrams per serving to ensure safe and responsible dosing!

YIELD: 2 CUPS, OR 16 OUNCES

CANNABIS-INFUSED OILS

In general, when it comes to baking and cooking, you cannot prepare most recipes without some sort of fat or oil. Cannabis-infused oil is one of the most important pantry staples you will make. When preparing this recipe at home, any oil will work; just be sure to check the different smoking/burning temperatures for each oil before you start cooking. Avocado oil is more neutral and versatile, but it's also considered a healthy fat. Canola oil is the most accessible, with a high smoking temperature. Olive oil is great for finishing a dish, such as when topping fresh pasta with a drizzle or for dipping bread. Sesame oil has more body and depth of flavor, which makes it perfect for Asian dishes such as poke and stir fry.

+ TARGET DOSE:

18.75 mg THC | 0 mg CBD per tablespoon

37.5 mg THC | 0 mg CBD per ounce

(You can always add more uninfused oil later to lower the dosage)

*These numbers will differ depending on the stain and source of the product you use. Refer to page 25 for at-home dosage calculations.

+ EQUIPMENT:

Digital scale

Silicone spatula

Tempered glass

Fine-mesh strainer

Parchment paper

+ INGREDIENTS:

3 grams decarboxylated flower of your choice

1 cup any oil (avocado, olive, sesame, canola, vegetable, coconut)

The Sous Vide Method

1. Fill the sous vide bag with the oil and decarboxylated flower, and then vacuum-seal it. If you don't have this setup, a freezer-grade sealable bag or mason jar will also work. Set your sous vide to 175°F (79°C).

2. When the water comes to temperature, place the bag inside the water bath for 4 hours. Remove the bag using tongs.

3. Pour the mixture over a cheesecloth-lined fine-mesh strainer, and voilá!

The Stovetop Method

1. Place the oil and decarboxylated flower in a saucepan with a thermometer. Begin to heat until it reaches 175°F to 200°F (79°C to 93°C).

2. Heat for 2 hours, constantly stirring and checking the temperature.

3. Line a fine-mesh strainer with cheesecloth, and strain into a tempered glass jar.

OR

1. Place the oil and decarboxylated flower in a mason jar with a lid.

2. Fill a saucepan with enough water to cover the infusion. Bring the water to temperature 200° (93°C), and place a towel at the bottom of the saucepan to protect the jar from touching the bottom of the pot.

3. Heat for 2 hours. Line a fine-mesh strainer with cheesecloth, and strain into a tempered glass jar.

> *Tip!* Oils, saturated fats, and butter can all interchangeably use various heating methods.

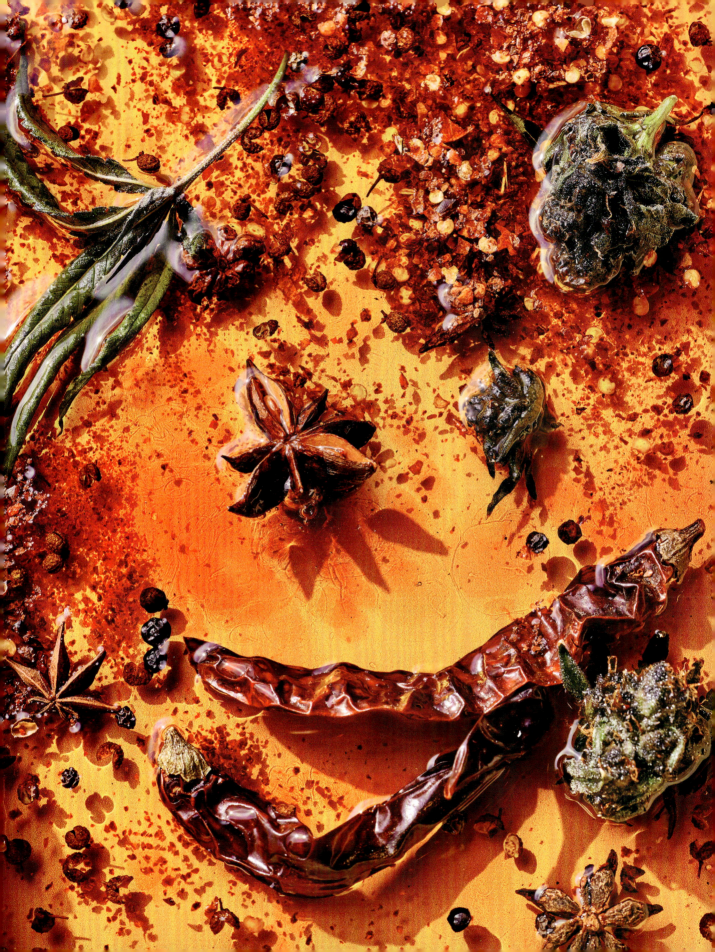

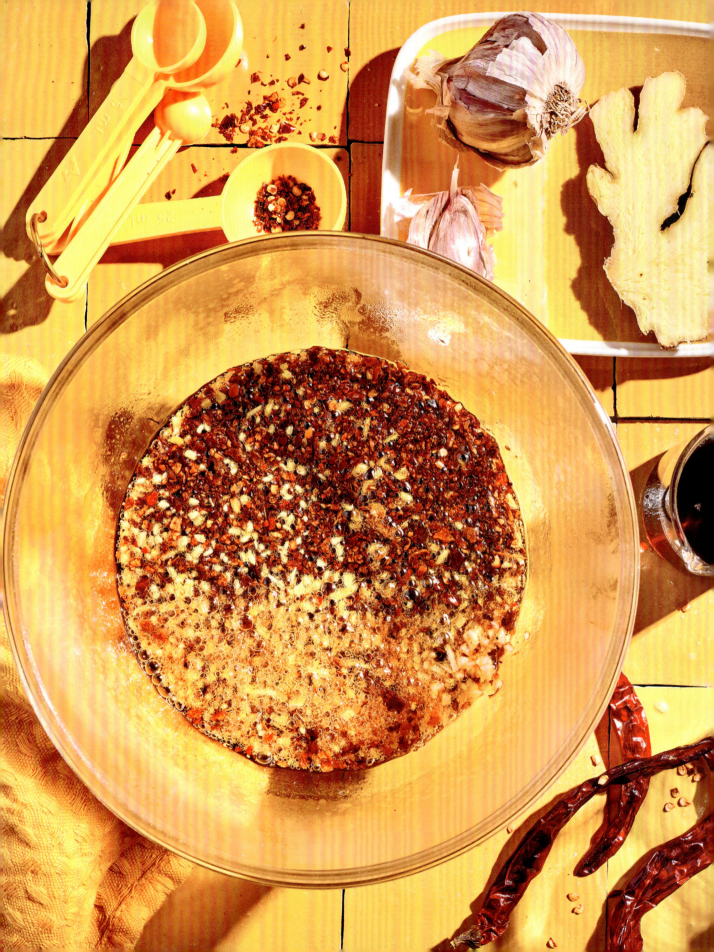

YIELD: 2 CUPS, OR 16 OUNCES

CANNABIS-INFUSED CHILI OIL

You can add chili oil to almost any dish you can think of. As many foodies would agree, a giant bowl of noodles isn't complete without a dollop of chili oil. The same can be true of dumplings, avocado toast, roasted veggies, vanilla ice cream (yes, you heard right!), and so much more. This recipe is one of the most basic and simple chili oils you can make, but no chili oil is the same. They can be very complex in flavor, with a multitude of ingredients and aromatics. Depending on the region, individual preference, and the dish, the range of possibilities and flavor profiles of chili oil is endless. Here's an easy but explosively delicious base chili oil, along with optional spices you can experiment with.

+ TARGET DOSE:

6.25 mg THC | 0 mg CBD per teaspoon

37.5 mg THC | 0 mg CBD per ounce

*These numbers will differ depending on the strain and source of the product you use. Refer to page 25 for at-home dosage calculations.

+ EQUIPMENT:

Digital scale

Food processor

Small saucepan

Coffee grinder (optional)

+ INGREDIENTS:

2 tablespoons garlic

1 tablespoon ginger

¼ teaspoon salt

½ cup chili flakes

¼ black or white pepper

1 cup avocado oil

1 cup Cannabis-Infused Sesame Oil (see page 44)

Optional spices: Korean flakes, Sichuan pepper flakes, star anise, cardamom, fermented black beans, shallots

1. Mince the garlic and ginger. In a tempered glass jar, combine the minced garlic and ginger with all the other dry ingredients.
2. Heat the avocado oil to just below smoking temperature, about 450°F (233°C); you want to make sure your oil is ripping hot.
3. Slowly pour the oil into the jar of ingredients little by little. **Caution:** As you do this, the ingredients will sizzle and can potentially boil over if the oil is poured too quickly; go slow and steady.
4. Give the jar a stir; then wait for it to cool to at least 200°F (93°C) before you pour in the cannabis-infused sesame oil.
5. Tighten the lid, and give it a couple shakes to incorporate everything. Then enjoy!

> *Tip!* We recommend using the infused sesame oil in this recipe. The other cup of noninfused vegetable oil should be used for the sizzling because you have to bring it to a high temperature. You do not want to use an infused oil for this because you'll burn off the terps and cannabinoids! If you have a coffee grinder handy, that can also work perfectly as a spice grinder. When buying whole spices, toasting and then grinding them on the spot while cooking is a great way to ensure that amazingly fresh and aromatic flavors appear in your dish.

YIELD: 2 CUPS, OR 16 OUNCES (4 STICKS)

CANNABIS-INFUSED BUTTER

This is the OG of edibles and cannabis cooking. You can't really go wrong with cannabis butter—infused baked potatoes, anyone? Whether you're using it to make rice cereal treats, baking a classic bud brownie, or simply spreading it on a piece of toasted sourdough with a pinch of Maldon salt, this iconic recipe is a must-have pantry item. It's undeniable that butter is one of *the* cheat staples of making anything taste more delicious, and this cannabis-infused butter is even more fantastic!

+ TARGET DOSE:

8 mg THC | 0 mg CBD per teaspoon

48 mg THC | 0 mg CBD per ounce

*These numbers will differ depending on the strain and source of the product you use. Refer to page 25 for at-home dosage calculations.

+ EQUIPMENT:

Digital scale
Thermometer
Measuring cups
Parchment paper
Saucepan
Tempered glass
Fine-mesh strainer
Cheesecloth
Freezer-grade sealable bags

+ INGREDIENTS:

16 ounces unsalted butter

4 grams decarboxylated flower of your choice

The Sous Vide Method

1. Fill the sous vide bag with unsalted butter and decarboxylated flower; then vacuum-seal it tight. If you don't have this setup, a freezer-grade sealable bag or mason jar will work just fine. Set your sous vide to 175°F (79°C).

2. When the water comes to temperature, place the bag inside the water bath for 4 hours.

3. Remove the bag using tongs. Pour the mixture over a cheesecloth-lined fine-mesh strainer into the storage container of your choice.

The Stovetop Method

1. Place the unsalted butter and decarboxylated flower in a saucepan with a thermometer. Begin to heat until it reaches 175°F to 200°F (79°C to 93°C).

2. Heat for 2 hours, constantly stirring and checking the temperature.

3. Line a fine-mesh strainer with cheesecloth, and strain into a tempered glass jar.

4. Let cool to room temperature; then store in the refrigerator until ready to use.

OR

1. Place the unsalted butter and decarboxylated flower in a mason jar. Seal tightly with a lid.

2. Fill a saucepan with enough water to cover the infusion. Begin to heat, bringing the temperature to 200°F (93°C).

3. Place a towel at the bottom of the saucepan to protect the jar from touching the bottom of the pot. Heat for 2 hours.

4. Line a fine-mesh strainer with cheesecloth, and strain into a tempered glass jar.

5. Let cool to room temperature; then store in the refrigerator until ready to use.

> *Tip!* If you want your infused butter to have a slightly longer shelf life, we recommend using clarified butter, or ghee, which is butter that has had the dairy removed from it, leaving only the fat. You can also make brown butter, straining out the dairy sediment before you start your infusion.

YIELD: 2 CUPS, OR 16 OUNCES

CANNABIS-INFUSED SATURATED FATS

We love to use good, hearty saturated fats when baking and cooking. Saturated fats are oils that solidify at room temperature. They add so much sweet, savory, or umami flavor to any dish where traditional oil is used. Saturated fats have a higher smoking point, but be careful not to overheat them and burn off any of that delicious cannabis infusion. Duck fat or bacon fat can be brushed on cornbread, grilled mushrooms, and roasted chicken; it can also be used as a spread for sandwiches, added to fried rice, and even blended into soups. Yum! Coconut oil is a game changer on popcorn, toasted nuts, granola, and glazed carrots; it can even be used for your hair and skin, as an infused topical.

+ TARGET DOSE:

8 mg THC | 0 mg CBD per teaspoon

50 mg THC | 0 mg CBD per ounce

*These numbers will differ depending on the strain and source of the product you use. Refer to page 25 for at-home dosage calculations.

+ EQUIPMENT:

Digital scale

Saucepan

Silicone spatula

Fine-mesh strainer

Tongs

Thermometer

Oven-safe glass jar

Foil

Deep hotel pan

Sous vide bag and vacuum sealer, or freezer-grade sealable bags

Sous vide machine

+ INGREDIENTS:

4 grams decarboxylated flower of your choice

1 cup duck fat or bacon fat

The Sous Vide Method

1. Measure out the decarboxylated flower.
2. Fill a sous vide bag with your saturated fat and decarboxylated flower, and then vacuum-seal it. If you don't have this setup, a freezer-grade sealable bag or mason jar will also work. Set your sous vide to 175°F (79°C).
3. When the water comes to temperature, place the bag inside the water bath for 4 hours. Remove the bag using tongs. Pour the mixture over a cheesecloth-lined fine-mesh strainer, and voilá!

The Oven Method

1. Set the oven to 200°F (93°C). Place your saturated fat and decarboxylated flower in a mason jar, and then cover it with foil.
2. Fill the hotel pan with enough water to submerge the jar just to the top of the ingredients. Place the lid of the jar inside the hotel pan so that the jar sits on top of it. (You can also use a towel.) This protects it from direct contact with the highest heat source.
3. Heat for 2 hours. Line a fine-mesh strainer with cheesecloth, and strain into a tempered glass jar.

> *Tip!* You can use numerous heating methods to create your infusion, as mentioned on page 42. Any of those methods work for creating oil-based infusions. Choose the one that seems the most approachable to you, in a timeframe that makes sense for your schedule and with the equipment you have access to. There's no wrong way to create these infusions, as long as you're staying on top of temperature control.

YIELD: 3 CUPS, OR 24 OUNCES

CANNABIS-INFUSED HONEY

Infused honey is one of the best and most versatile staples to have in your pantry. Drizzle it into your salad dressings, marinades, sauces, or beverages, or enjoy it as a condiment for your charcuterie board as a dose-yourself option for guests next time you're hosting. When it comes to cannabis-infused honey, the combinations are endless! When preparing this recipe, things can get a little sticky. Keeping your work area clean and tidy as you go is a great way to minimize the mess.

+ TARGET DOSE:

4 mg THC | 0 mg CBD per teaspoon

25 mg THC | 0 mg CBD per ounce

*These numbers will differ depending on the strain and source of the product you use. Refer to page 25 for at-home dosage calculations.

+ EQUIPMENT:

Digital scale

Saucepan

Silicone spatula

Cheesecloth

Fine-mesh strainer

Tempered glass container with lid

Thermometer

+ INGREDIENTS:

3 grams decarboxylated flower of your choice

1 cup honey

1. Weigh out the decarboxylated cannabis. In a saucepan, using a thermometer, heat the honey to 170°F (77°C). Then stir in the cannabis.
2. Simmer over low heat for 1 hour, constantly stirring and checking the temperature.
3. Line a fine-mesh strainer with cheesecloth, and pour the infused honey into the tempered glass jar with lid.

> *Tip!* Shake or stir your infusion vigorously as it cools down in 10°F increments. This will help ensure emulsification.

YIELD: 2 CUPS, OR 16 OUNCES

CANNABIS-INFUSED SUGAR

This infusion recipe is ideal for any dish that calls for sugar. Cannabis-infused sugar will be one of the easiest infusions to incorporate in your daily life, such as a little in your cup of coffee or tea in the morning as a nice way to wake and bake. You can also take your hosting game to the next level with an infused sugar-rimmed cocktail, or grind your infused sugar into a powdered sugar to dust on sweet treats. Most types of sugar will work in this recipe, except for artificial sweeteners. These have different stabilizers and additives that could negatively impact the results of your recipe, so it's best to use natural sugars.

+ TARGET DOSE:

5 mg THC | 0 mg CBD per ¼ teaspoon

250 mg THC | 0 mg CBD per cup

*These numbers will differ depending on the strain and source of the product you use. Refer to page 25 for at-home dosage calculations.

+ EQUIPMENT:

Digital scale

Measuring cups

Parchment paper

Glass bowl or glass baking dish (the more surface room to spread out the sugar, the faster it will dry)

Cheesecloth

Silicone spatula

Airtight glass container

+ INGREDIENTS:

3½ ounces Cannabis-Infused Alcohol Tincture (see page 58)

2 cups granulated sugar (or turbinado sugar, or sugar of your choice)

1. Prepare the alcohol tincture recipe on page 58.

2. Pour the sugar into the glass container, followed by the cannabis tincture. Stir well with a silicone spatula, making sure all the sugar granules are thoroughly coated in the tincture. Make sure it is evenly spread for drying.

3. Cover with cheesecloth, and secure with a rubber band or string. Airflow is super important in this process, so be sure not to cover the dish with a lid. Place in a dry, unbothered area where this mixture can air-dry for about 2 to 3 days; gently stir each day. Depending on the humidity and weather in your region, the timing may vary. When all the moisture from the alcohol has completely evaporated and the consistency is similar to the kind of sugar you started with, you know that it's done. Store in a dry, airtight container.

> *Tip!* **Throughout this book, several recipes call for cannabis-infused powdered sugar. To create, simply follow this recipe as directed, then grind the infused sugar into a fine dust before using. Due to the nature of sugar and alcohol, the pantry life of this infusion is fairly long.**

YIELD: 1 CUP, OR 8 OUNCES (PEANUT OIL) | YIELD: 2½ CUPS, OR 20 OUNCES (PEANUT BUTTER)

HOW TO MAKE HASH-INFUSED PEANUT OIL & PEANUT BUTTER

If you're a fan of peanut butter, you're going to love making hash-infused peanut butter! The best way to create this recipe at home is using ice water hash for the infusion. Because you're making peanut butter, it's best to infuse the recipe using peanut oil, which you can source from your local grocery store. The ice water hash and peanut oil flavors work well together, plus the hash allows for a more potent infusion to best enhance this recipe. We recommend adding a dash of salt and a bit of honey to complement the flavor. It's the perfect addition to Peanut Butter & Jelly and beyond!

+ TARGET DOSE:

1000 mg THC | 0 mg CBD per cup

125 mg THC | 0 mg CBD per ⅛ cup or per ounce

21 mg THC | 0 mg CBD per teaspoon

+ EQUIPMENT:

Clear baking dish

Aluminum foil

Two 8-ounce tempered glass Mason jars

Saucepan

Thermometer

Oven mitt

Fine-mesh strainer

Cheesecloth

Blender or food processor

+ INGREDIENTS:

For the Peanut Oil:

2 grams ice water hash of your choice (using 50 percent THC content or higher per gram)

1 cup (218 grams) peanut oil

For the Peanut Butter:

24 ounces (679.50 grams) unsalted dry-roasted peanuts

⅛ cup ice water hash–infused peanut oil

Dash of salt and honey

For the Peanut Oil:

1. The first step is to decarboxylate the hash. Preheat the oven to 200°F (93°C).
2. Transfer the hash to a clear baking dish, cover with aluminum foil, and place it into the oven. Bake for 30 to 40 minutes; then remove from heat.
3. In an 8-ounce (240 mL) *tempered glass* mason jar, combine the ice water hash with 1 cup peanut oil. Stir to combine, and then seal the top tightly.
4. Fill the bottom of a small saucepan with water.
5. Set the mason jar inside, and begin to heat over medium-low heat; the water should not go to the top of the mason jar.
6. Continue to heat until you reach around 200°F (93°C). Heat for 1 hour, making sure the water does not exceed 211°F (99°C). Check frequently, and refill the saucepan with water as needed due to evaporation.
7. When finished, remove the mason jar safely using an oven mitt, and let the jar cool. If any hash debris is floating in the oil, filter it through a fine-mesh strainer lined with cheesecloth into a sterilized 8-ounce (240 mL) mason jar. The peanut oil will stay fresh for several months if it's stored properly in a cool, dark cabinet.

* Recipe continued on page 55

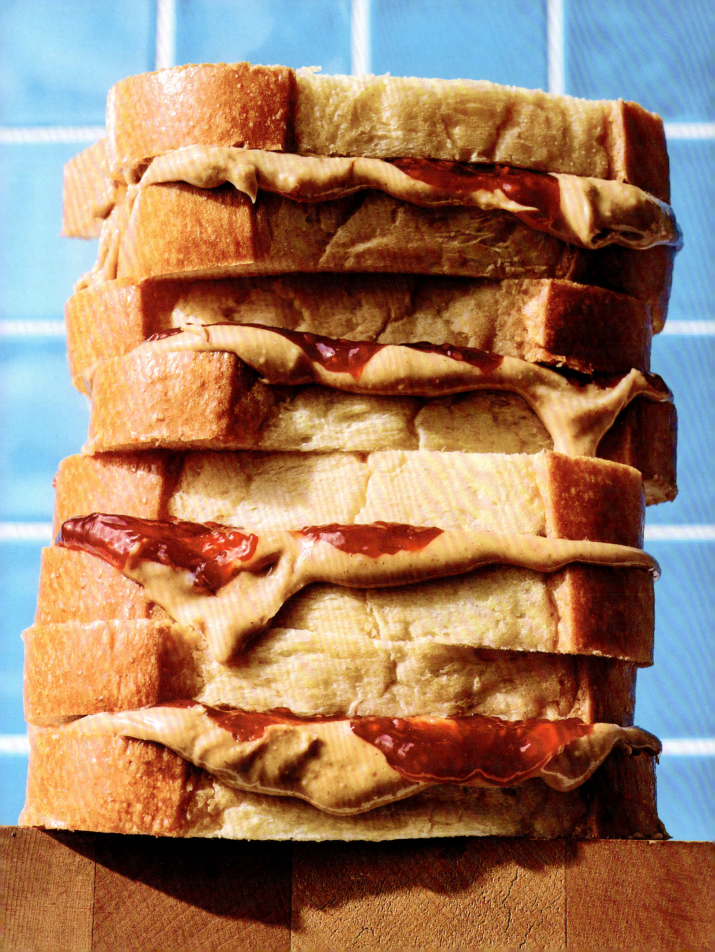

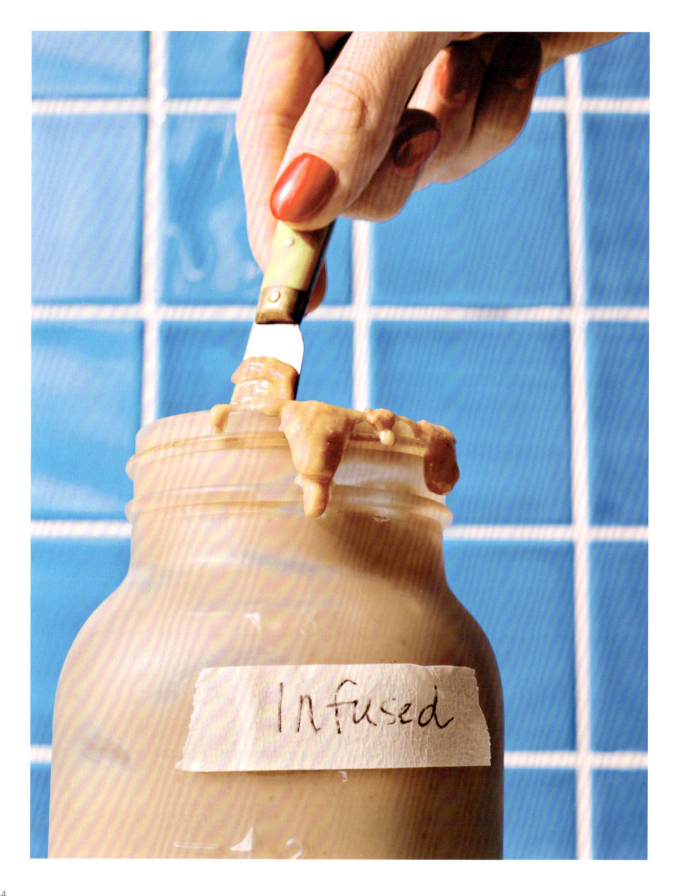

For the Peanut Butter:

1. Add the unsalted dry-roasted peanuts to the bottom of a food processor. Blend on high for 5 to 8 minutes. During this process, the peanuts will turn into ground pieces and then begin to clump together and break down into a smoother consistency.

2. When the texture is creamy (but not liquefied!) add ⅛ cup of the ice water hash–infused peanut oil, and continue to blend until combined well. Add a dash of salt and honey to taste; then blend again.

3. Transfer the cannabis-infused peanut butter into a storage container of your choice, and enjoy!

> *Tip!* **When blending the peanuts, be careful not to over blend as this can impact your peanut butter's texture making it overly liquified. Keep a close eye during this process, and if you prefer a chunkier peanut butter, blend until your desired texture is achieved.**

YIELD: 2½ CUPS, OR 20 OUNCES

CANNABIS-INFUSED BITTERS

If you like making cocktails, cannabis-infused bitters is a fantastic ingredient you can use to enhance a variety of mixed drinks. Not only do bitters act as a flavoring agent to blend the ingredients in a drink, but they also add unique aromas and flavors, making the beverage even more complex. When preparing bitters at home, the key ingredient to source is the actual bittering agent itself (cinchona bark, horehound, wild cherry bark, and so on). All of these bittering agents come from plants and are typically sourced from bark, roots, or dried herbs. When combining bittering agents with herbal products, you can select the type that best pairs with your cannabis's aromas and flavors. For this recipe, you'll be using a combination of horehound and cinchona bark, which are well balanced and pair exceptionally well with blood orange and spicy notes. The following are two methods for preparing cannabis-infused bitters at home. Always remember to sample your bitters before combining into a beverage, to best gauge the potency.

+ TARGET DOSE:

3 mg THC | < 1 mg CBD per ¼ teaspoon or 2 dashes (12 to 16 drops)

62 mg THC | 3 mg CBD per ounce

*These numbers will differ depending on the strain and source of the product you use. Refer to page 25 for at-home dosage calculations.

+ EQUIPMENT:

One 32-ounce (940 mL) sterilized mason jar

Two 16-ounce (480 mL) sterilized mason jars

One 8-ounce (240 mL) sterilized mason jar

Cheesecloth

Fine-mesh strainer

Airtight swing bottle or amber bottle with a dropper cap

+ INGREDIENTS:

10 grams decarboxylated flower of your choice

⅓ cup dried blood orange peels

5 whole allspice berries

1 cinnamon stick

1 (1-inch) piece fresh ginger, peeled and sliced into pieces

¼ teaspoon cinchona bark

½ teaspoon horehound

2 cups high-proof vodka (80 proof or higher)

¾ cup water

½ ounce noninfused simple syrup (optional)

Tip! If blood oranges are out of season, simply swap for regular dried orange peels, which you can source online or make at home.

Tip! To create the best bitters, make sure all your ingredients are fully submerged into the vodka or spirit you're working with. If you need more than 2 cups, feel free to top off the jar, ensuring that everything is immersed into the liquid.

1. Using a 32-ounce (940 mL) mason jar, add the decarboxylated cannabis flower, dried blood orange peels, allspice, cinnamon stick, ginger, and bittering agents to the bottom of the jar.
2. Top with high-proof vodka, seal with an airtight lid, and shake vigorously.
3. Steep this mixture for 10 days, stored in a dark cabinet. Be sure to shake daily for the best extraction.
4. When the 10 days are up, separate the solids from the liquids over a clean 16-ounce (480 mL) mason jar using a fine-mesh strainer and cheesecloth. Seal the mason jar filled with the filtered infused bitters, and store it in a dark cabinet until further use. If you want stronger-tasting and more potent bitters, follow the steps as directed, but infuse for 2 weeks or more. Just be sure to keep checking on flavor/potency until you find your preferred style of bitters.

To dilute the bitters (optional based on taste preference, or if using a high-proof spirit [120 proof or more]):

1. Follow the previous steps. Then after filtering, transfer the solids into a saucepan and top with ¾ cup (175 mL) water. Heat over medium heat for 5 to 6 minutes.
2. Remove from heat, and let cool. When the mixture reaches room temperature, transfer it to a clean 16-ounce (480 mL) mason jar, and steep for 3 days in the refrigerator, agitating daily.
3. When the 3 days are up, separate the liquid from the solids using a fine-mesh strainer and cheesecloth into a clean 8-ounce (240 mL) mason jar; discard the solids/sediment. For the best clarity, filter a few times to remove all leftover debris.
4. Add this liquid mixture to the infused vodka that you've already created, and then add the simple syrup (if using).
5. Shake well. Let the bitters rest for a few additional days, allowing any leftover sediment to sink to the bottom of the mason jar.
6. When ready, carefully filter out the clean liquid resting on top using a fine-mesh strainer and cheesecloth. Leave the sediment behind; then discard.
7. To best preserve your bitters, transfer the liquid into dark glassware or amber glass bottles. Store at room temperature in a dark cabinet for several months.

The Heated Sous Vide Method

1. Similar to creating an alcohol tincture (page 58), using the sous vide to prepare cannabis-infused bitters is the fastest and safest way to create this type of infusion with heat.
2. To prepare at home, set your sous vide bath to 140°F (60°C).
3. Combine the decarboxylated cannabis flower, dried blood orange peels, allspice, cinnamon, ginger, bittering agents, and high-proof vodka in a tempered glass mason jar (seal tight!) or an airtight vacuum-seal pouch (only if using a chamber vacuum sealer—otherwise, you'll lose liquid, and the pouch might not seal).
4. Place the pouch or jar into the sous vide bath, and heat for 2 hours. Using an oven mitt or tongs, remove from heat; then let cool to room temperature.
5. Separate the solids from the liquids over a clean 16-ounce (480 mL) mason jar using a fine-mesh strainer and cheesecloth.
6. Seal the mason jar filled with the filtered infused vodka, and store it in a dark cabinet until further use.
7. To dilute, follow the instructions above.

YIELD: 1 CUP, OR 8 OUNCES

CANNABIS-INFUSED ALCOHOL TINCTURE

Whether you're cooking or mixing up a tasty beverage, having a cannabis-infused alcohol tincture on hand is a great way to enhance just about any liquid-based recipe. Using a high-proof grain alcohol for the extraction (clocking in at 120 proof or higher), the following techniques will allow you to capture a full spectrum of cannabis compounds for the most potent infusion. If you don't currently own a sous vide, you can easily prepare this recipe using the freezer method, which requires only a few ingredients and minimal equipment. By freezing the tincture during the extraction process, you're preventing pronounced green, herbaceous notes from tainting the tincture. In the end, this delivers a cleaner flavor. When adding this potent tincture to drinks, measure in milliliters using a precise dropper with measurements. Because you'll need only a very small amount to infuse the drink, you won't taste the alcohol or feel its effects (this is the goal). You should feel only the cannabis effects, unless you're mixing up a cocktail that contains additional alcohol. Always remember to sample your tincture before combining into a beverage, to best gauge the potency. Here are two ways to prepare a cannabis-infused tincture at home.

+ TARGET DOSE:

5 mg THC | < 1 mg CBD per milliliter

145 mg THC | 10 mg CBD per ounce

*These numbers will differ depending on the strain and source of the product you use. Refer to page 25 for at-home dosage calculations.

+ INGREDIENTS:

9 grams decarboxylated flower of your choice

1 cup (240 mL) high-proof clear grain alcohol (120 proof or higher)

+ EQUIPMENT:

16-ounce mason jar

Fine-mesh strainer

Cheesecloth

Airtight storage container of your choice, or split between amber glass bottles with dropper caps

The Freezer Method

1. Combine 9 grams of decarboxylated flower with 1 cup (240 mL) high-proof clear grain alcohol in a mason jar. Seal the jar tightly, and place it in the freezer for 10 days. Shake the jar every day to help with the extraction process.
2. After the 10 days, line a fine-mesh strainer with cheesecloth, and filter out the solids from the infused alcohol.
3. Store in an airtight container of your choice or in amber glass bottles with dropper caps. For best results, filter a few times to help with clarity. Store in the refrigerator for several months.

The Heated Method

1. Using a sous vide to heat during the extraction process is the fastest way to create a cannabis-infused alcohol tincture. Instead of waiting 10 days, you can create this infusion within 2 hours! The sous vide is also the safest heating method to use; you should never heat alcohol over a gas stove or open flame and stay far below 170°F (77°C) as alcohol is flammable at this point.
2. To prepare at home, set your sous vide bath to 140°F (60°C).
3. Combine 1 cup high-proof clear grain alcohol with 9 grams of decarboxylated cannabis into a tempered glass mason jar (seal tight!) or an airtight vacuum-seal pouch (only if using a chamber vacuum sealer—otherwise, you'll lose liquid, and the pouch might not seal).
4. Place the jar or pouch into the sous vide bath and heat for 2 hours.
5. Using an oven mitt or tongs, remove from heat; let cool to room temperature.
6. Line a fine-mesh strainer with cheesecloth, and strain into an airtight container of your choice or amber glass bottles with dropper caps. For the best clarity, filter a few times to remove all flower debris. Store in the refrigerator for several months.

> *Tip!* If you decide to use the heated method to prepare the tincture, keep in mind that it will have a much darker color and stronger cannabis notes, compared to the freezer method (not as clean looking/tasting because heat accelerates the extraction of everything, including chlorophyll). However, this process produces faster and more potent results if you're in need of a quick infusion.

YIELD: JUST OVER 2 CUPS, OR 17 OUNCES

CANNABIS-INFUSED SIMPLE SYRUP

When preparing any beverage at home, one of the most versatile ingredients to have on hand is a cannabis-infused simple syrup. Acting as a sweetener for your recipes, infused simple syrup blends seamlessly into any liquid-based recipe and can be enhanced with a number of herbs and spices to boost the flavor of the drink. Here are a few ways to prepare this recipe at home, using a combination of water and granulated sugar. If you prefer to use a different sugar base, such as honey, simply swap the sugar in the recipe for 1 cup (340 grams) honey, and follow the directions as noted. Always remember to sample your simple syrup before you combine it into a beverage, to best gauge the potency.

+ TARGET DOSE:

20 to 21 mg THC | 1.5 mg CBD per ounce

10 to 11 mg THC | < 1 mg CBD per half ounce

*These numbers will differ depending on the strain and source of the product you use. Refer to page 25 for at-home dosage calculations.

+ EQUIPMENT:

Digital scale

Saucepan

Silicone spatula

Measuring cups

Thermometer

Cheesecloth

Fine-mesh strainer

Airtight storage container of your choice

+ INGREDIENTS:

2.5 to 4 grams decarboxylated flower of your choice (use 4 grams for a stronger dose)

2 cups (480 mL) water

2 cups (400 grams) granulated sugar

1½ tablespoons (22.5 mL) food-grade vegetable glycerin

1. Weigh out the decarboxylated cannabis, and set aside.
2. Add the water and sugar to a small saucepan over medium heat. Stir until the granulated sugar dissolves completely into the water.
3. Reduce the heat to 160°F to 180°F (71°C to 82°C). Add the decarboxylated cannabis and vegetable glycerin, and stir to combine.
4. Simmer over low heat for 1 hour, occasionally stirring, scraping the sides of the pan to remove flower and sugar debris. Remove from heat.
5. Line a fine-mesh strainer with cheesecloth, and pour the infused simple syrup into the container of your choice to separate out the solids. For the best clarity, filter the simple syrup a few times through the cheesecloth to catch all leftover debris. Let cool, then store in the refrigerator until further use. Always shake before serving.

Cannabis-Infused Mint Simple Syrup

1. To create mint-infused simple syrup, follow the previous steps, but add 1 cup (96 grams) mint leaves to the saucepan after the sugar dissolves into the water.
2. Massage the mint leaves with your hands to release the oils before adding them into the saucepan with the decarboxylated cannabis.
3. Follow the directions above, and be sure to filter through cheesecloth and a fine-mesh strainer to remove the solids. Store in the refrigerator for up to 3 weeks.

> *Tip!* If you want to add some spicy notes to your drinks, simply swap the mint for either 4 sticks of cinnamon, 1 tablespoon cracked cardamom, 1 tablespoon whole allspice, or 3 whole nutmegs (or a combination of spices); then follow the directions as listed.

YIELD: ABOUT 1½ CUPS, OR 12 OUNCES

CANNABIS-INFUSED COCONUT MILK

As a perfect ingredient to add to piña coladas and other tropical drinks, coconut milk is easy to infuse, plus it's an ideal extraction ingredient with its high fat content. If you're not a fan of coconut milk, you can swap it for dairy milk or soy milk—just be sure it's rich enough with healthy fat to absorb as many cannabis compounds as possible. Remember to sample your infused coconut milk before combining into a beverage, to best gauge the potency.

+ TARGET DOSE:

18 to 19 mg THC | 1 mg CBD per ounce

9 to 10 mg THC | < 1 mg CBD per half-ounce

*These numbers will differ depending on the strain and source of the product you use. Refer to page 25 for at-home dosage calculations (and be sure to factor in 20 to 25 percent loss of liquid due to evaporation)

+ INGREDIENTS:

1.5 to 3 grams decarboxylated flower of your choice (use 3 grams for a stronger dose, but it will taste/look greener)

2 cups (480 mL) unsweetened coconut milk (or milk of your choice)

+ EQUIPMENT:

Digital scale

Measuring cups

Small saucepan

Thermometer

Silicone spatula

Cheesecloth

Fine-mesh strainer

Airtight storage container of your choice

1. Weigh out the decarboxylated flower. Set aside.
2. Add the coconut milk to a saucepan over medium heat. Heat to 160°F to 180°F (71°C to 82°C), and then add the decarboxylated cannabis. Stir to combine.
3. Keep a close eye on the temperature, stirring frequently and scraping the sides of the saucepan to remove any flower debris.
4. After 1 hour of cooking, remove the infused coconut milk from heat. Some of the milk will evaporate, so you will have less than your original 2 cups.
5. Using a cheesecloth and fine-mesh strainer, strain the infused coconut milk into an airtight container of your choice for storage. Let cool, and then put it in the fridge to chill before serving.

> *Tip!* For this recipe, you'll want to use unsweetened coconut milk that's meant to be refrigerated and won't solidify when chilled. Choose a coconut milk that's available in the refrigerated milk section at your local grocery store instead of using canned coconut milk.

How to Make Cannabis-Infused Coconut Cream

To prepare on the stove, follow the previous steps and swap coconut milk for unsweetened coconut cream. **Important!** Make sure to place the decarboxylated cannabis in an all-natural tea bag for this infusion, otherwise, the flower solids and particles will have a difficult time filtering out because the cream can be thick as the milk evaporates with heat! If the coconut cream you're using is solidified, simply add it to the saucepan and heat until it liquifies; then follow the directions as noted. Although the stovetop method works for this infusion, we highly recommend using a sous vide, if you have one, to avoid evaporation. Here are the directions:

1. Set your sous vide bath to 160°F (71°C).
2. Combine the decarboxylated cannabis flower with the unsweetened coconut cream in a tempered glass mason jar (seal tight!) or an airtight vacuum-seal pouch (only if using a chamber vacuum sealer—otherwise, you'll lose liquid, and the pouch might not seal).
3. Place the jar or pouch into the sous vide bath, and heat for 2 hours. Using an oven mitt or tongs, remove from heat. Let cool to room temperature.
4. Separate the solids from the liquids over a clean 16-ounce (480 mL) mason jar, using a fine-mesh strainer and cheesecloth.
5. Seal the mason jar filled with the filtered unsweetened coconut cream, and store it in the refrigerator until ready to use.

YIELD: JUST OVER 2 CUPS, OR 17 OUNCES

CANNABIS-INFUSED FRUIT SYRUP

When summer berries are in season, making a cannabis-infused fruit syrup is a delicious way to infuse cocktails, mocktails, and even vinaigrette dressings! This colorful and flavorful pantry item is easy to make and versatile, depending on what fruit is available and in season. This recipe is made in a similar way as cannabis-infused simple syrup (page 60), but with a few extra steps.

+ TARGET DOSE:

20 to 21 mg THC | 1.5 mg CBD per ounce

10 to 11 mg THC | < 1 mg CBD per half-ounce

*These numbers will differ depending on the strain and source of the product you use. Refer to page 25 for at-home dosage calculations.

+ EQUIPMENT:

Digital scale

Saucepan

Silicone spatula

Potato masher or fork

Measuring cups

Cheesecloth

Fine-mesh strainer

Thermometer

Airtight storage container of your choice

+ INGREDIENTS:

2.5 to 4 grams decarboxylated flower of your choice (use 4 grams for a stronger dose, but it will taste greener)

2 cups (480 mL) water

2 cups (400 grams) granulated sugar

2 cups fresh raspberries (see note)

1½ tablespoons (22.5 mL) food-grade vegetable glycerin

Recipe continued on page 67

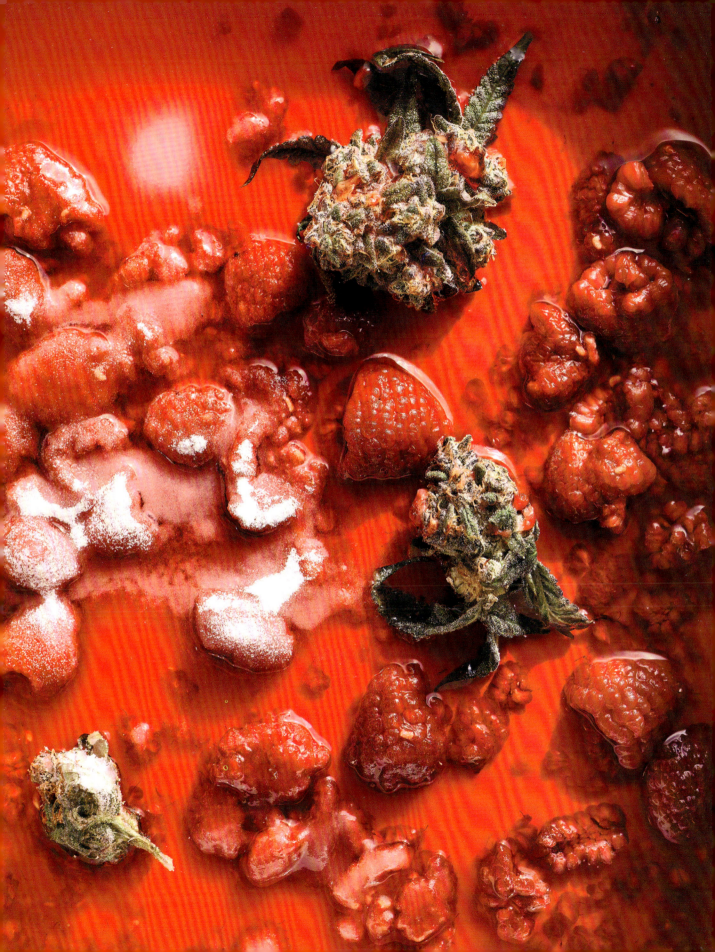

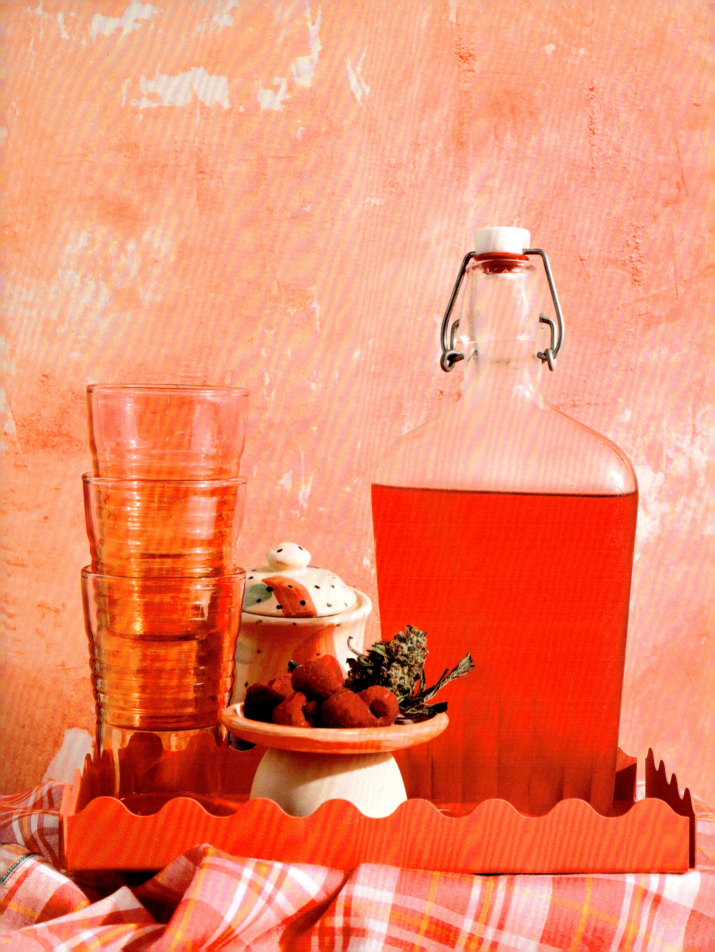

1. Weigh out the decarboxylated cannabis, and set aside.
2. In a small saucepan, bring the water and sugar to a soft boil, stirring occasionally until the sugar dissolves.
3. Remove from heat, and stir in the raspberries. When the raspberries have warmed up, use a fork or potato masher to mash the raspberries into a pulp.
4. Cover the saucepan, and steep for 1 hour. Strain through a fine-mesh strainer lined with cheesecloth.
5. Transfer the fruit syrup to a clean saucepan, and heat to 160°F to 180°F (71°C to 82°C). Add the decarboxylated cannabis and vegetable glycerin; stir to combine.
6. Simmer over low heat for 1 hour, occasionally stirring, scraping the sides of the pan to remove flower debris. Remove from heat.
7. Line a fine-mesh strainer with cheesecloth; then pour the infused fruit syrup into the container of your choice to separate out the solids. For the best clarity, filter the syrup a few times through the cheesecloth to catch all leftover debris.
8. Let cool, and store in the refrigerator until further use. Always shake before serving.

> *Tip!* **Depending on what berries are in season, you can easily swap raspberries for blackberries or strawberries (or a combination of all three!). Follow the directions as listed, and then combine into your favorite drinks or vinaigrette.**
>
> *Tip!* **For a burst of berry freshness, prepare this recipe using a cannabis strain that presents berry notes, such as Sunset Sherbet, Berry White, or Strawberry Cough.**

YIELD: ABOUT 2 CUPS, OR 16 OUNCES

FAT-WASHED INFUSIONS TWO WAYS

If you've ever tasted bacon-flavored vodka or olive oil–infused gin, you've most likely come across a fat-washed spirit. In the mixology world, *fat washing* is a method of infusion that relies on the extraction that occurs between fat flavor compounds and alcohol. Spirits are best for this method because they have the ability to extract and dissolve fatty flavors into the liquid, leaving behind mouthwatering fat-flavored alcohol. When combined with cannabis, fat washing is a successful extraction technique because THC, CBD, and other cannabis compounds love binding with fat-based *and* alcohol-based solutions. This process allows these compounds to be extracted and infused into the spirit you're working with, creating a delicious, smooth, and creamy alcohol base for infused cocktails. Here are two ways to create fat-washed infusions at home using bourbon and rum.

+ TARGET DOSE:

For Brown Butter–Washed Bourbon :

6 mg THC | 0 mg CBD per ounce

3 mg THC | 0 mg CBD per ½ ounce

96 mg THC | 0 mg CBD total

For Coconut-Washed Rum:

9.4 mg THC | 0 mg CBD per ounce

4.7 mg THC | 0 mg CBD per ½ ounce

150 mg THC | 0 mg CBD total

*Because these infusions are combined with alcohol and intended to be used in a cocktail, it's best to stay below 10 mg THC per ounce so you don't overdo it (flip to page 29 for tips on mixing cannabis with alcohol). These numbers will differ depending on the strain and source of the product you use. Refer to page 25 for at-home dosage calculations.

+ EQUIPMENT:

For Brown Butter–Washed Bourbon:

Sauté pan

Silicone spatula

One 32-ounce (940 mL) sterilized mason jar

Fine-mesh strainer

Cheesecloth

One 16-ounce (480 mL) sterilized mason jar or airtight swing-top bottle

For Coconut-Washed Rum:

One 32-ounce (940 mL) sterilized mason jar

Fine-mesh strainer

Cheesecloth

One 16-ounce (480 mL) sterilized mason jar or airtight swing-top bottle

+ INGREDIENTS:

For Brown Butter–Washed Bourbon:

½ cup (112.5 grams, or 1 stick) cannabis-infused butter (see page 48)

2 cups (480 mL) bourbon

For Coconut-Washed Rum:

2 cups (480 mL) rum

½ cup (108 grams) liquified cannabis-infused coconut oil (see page 44)

For Brown Butter–Washed Bourbon:

1. Using a light-colored sauté pan, begin to melt the canna-butter over medium/low heat, stirring frequently.
2. Continue to move the butter around until it begins to foam and turn golden brown (it should smell nutty). Be very careful not to boil or burn the butter (keep the temperature at or below 250°F [121°C]) to protect the cannabis compounds and the butter.
3. Remove from heat, let cool, and then transfer to a 32-ounce (940 mL) sterilized mason jar.
4. Add the bourbon, and shake the two ingredients together vigorously. Cool to room temperature; then place in the freezer for 24 hours (or until the fat solidifies at the top of the mason jar).
5. Remove from the freezer, poke a hole through the side of the solidified butter, and then strain the liquid through a fine-mesh strainer lined with cheesecloth to catch any leftover solids and debris. Repeat until the liquid contains no solids.
6. Transfer to a clean 16-ounce (480 mL) sterilized mason jar or airtight swing-top bottle, and store in the refrigerator for up to 2 weeks. You might need to filter again as the butter particles resolidify.

> *Tip!* Brown butter–washed bourbon is decadent, perfectly combining buttery and nutty flavors into a number of craft cocktails. Flip to page 132 for a Brown Butter Old Fashioned.

For Coconut-Washed Rum:

1. In a 32-ounce (940 mL) sterilized mason jar, add the liquified cannabis-infused coconut oil; top with rum. Shake the jar vigorously until well combined; then place in the freezer for 24 hours (or until the coconut oil solidifies at the top of the mason jar).
2. Remove from the freezer, poke a hole through the side of the solidified coconut oil, and strain the liquid through a fine-mesh strainer lined with cheesecloth to catch any leftover solids and debris. Repeat until the liquid contains no solids.
3. Transfer to a clean 16-ounce (480 mL) sterilized mason jar or airtight swing-top bottle, and store in the refrigerator for up to 2 weeks. You might need to filter again if the coconut oil continues to solidify and separate from the rum.

> *Tip!* This delicious fat-washed infusion is perfect for adding to piña coladas (see page 127) and a number of tiki drinks, or any recipe that could use a hint of tropical flavor!

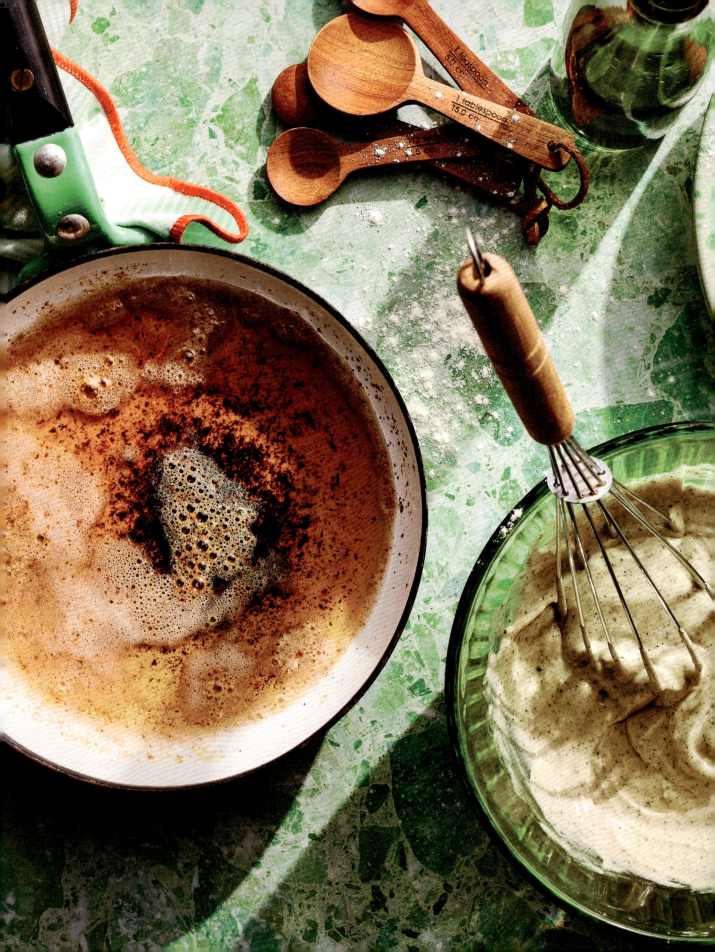

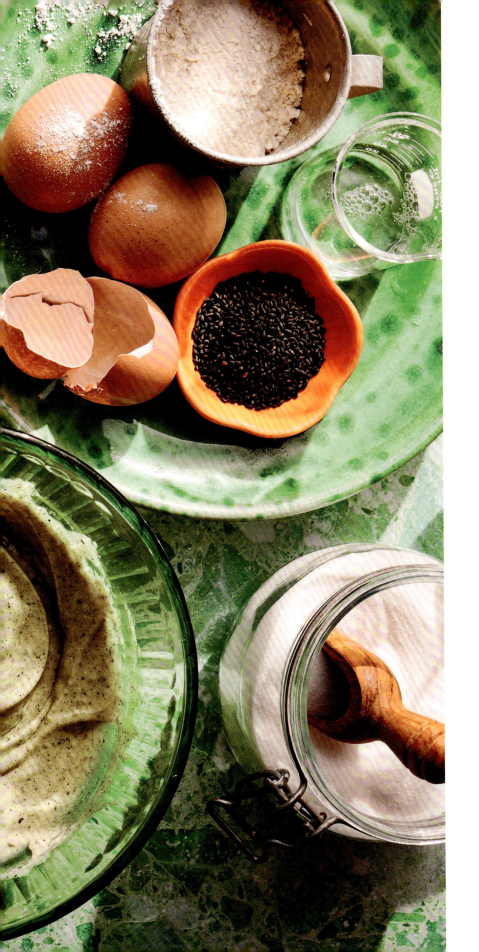

THE RECIPES

CHAPTER 3

Now let's dig into the recipes! Throughout this chapter, you will find a selection of delicious eats and drinks that will satisfy every craving, including baked sweets, savory eats, cannabis drinks, and noninfused munchies. Keep in mind, the target dosage listed in each recipe can be a reference point for your infusions, but your final outcome will vary depending on the cannabis item you've infused it with. Always be sure to calculate the estimated dosage per serving and consume responsibly. We hope you enjoy this collection of some of our favorite flavors!

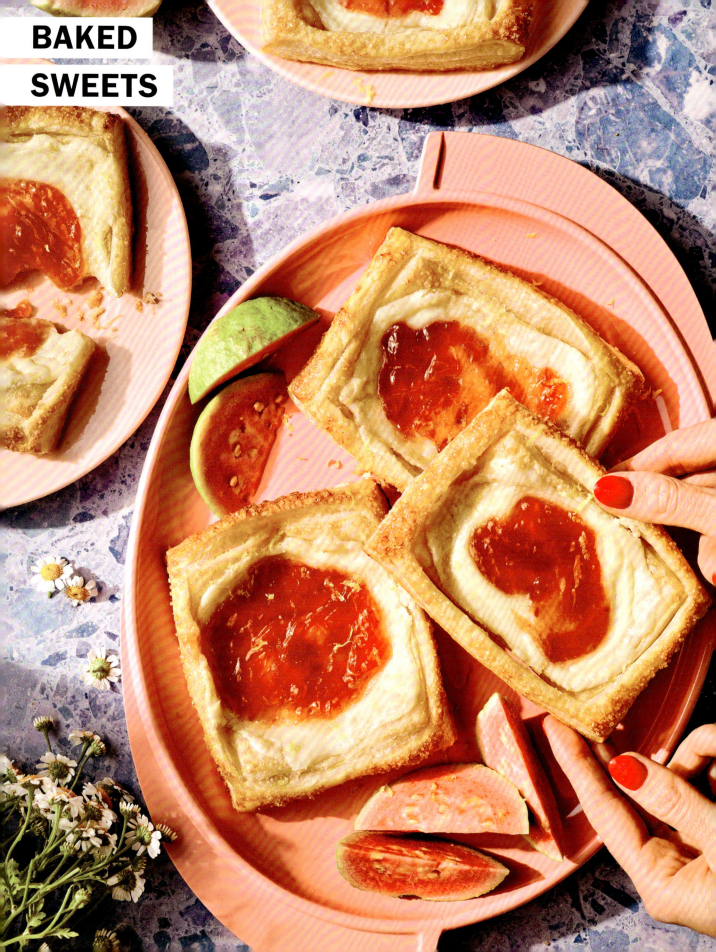

BAKED SWEETS

YIELD: 6 PASTRIES

GUAVA CREAM CHEESE PASTRY WITH SALTED EGG YOLK

Guava cream cheese? Yes, please! This delicious pastry recipe is about to become your new go-to recipe for brunch, picnics, daytime gatherings, or anytime you get a craving when your favorite local patisserie is closed. Elevated, multilayered, yet simple to make, this delicious treat has flaky layers of puff pastry with sweet guava filling and gooey cream cheese that contrasts with a sprinkle of rich salted egg yolk for a hint of savory. This dish is truly indulgent. Sprinkle as much or as little cannabis-infused sugar on the edges as you like!

+ TARGET DOSE:

Your preferred dose (using cannabis-infused turbinado sugar, page 51)

+ EQUIPMENT:

Baking sheet

Parchment paper

Whisk

Measuring spoon

Silicone brush

+ INGREDIENTS:

4 ounces cream cheese, at room temperature

¼ cup powdered sugar, divided

¼ teaspoon maple syrup

1 sheet puff pastry, thawed

¼ cup guava jam

1 egg

Salted egg yolk

Cannabis-infused turbinado sugar for the edges, at your preferred dosage

1. Preheat the oven to 425°F (218°C), and line a baking sheet with parchment paper.
2. Whip the cream cheese with ¼ cup powdered sugar and the maple syrup.
3. Lay out the defrosted puff pastry sheet, and cut it into 6 equal rectangles.
4. Using a paring knife, cut a ½-inch border around the puff pastry.
5. Spread a thin layer of whipped cream cheese inside the inner border of the puff pastry.
6. Spoon the guava jam on top of the cream cheese.
7. Beat one egg as an egg wash, and brush the egg wash onto the outer edges of the puff pastry.
8. Sprinkle the egg-washed edges with turbinado sugar and grated salted egg yolk.
9. Place the pastries on the middle rack in the oven, and bake for 12 to 15 minutes until they're golden brown and flakey.

Tip! We love the sweet guava in this pastry, but if you can't find guava jam, you can substitute with any fruit jam, such as apricot, strawberry, or even orange marmalade. Avoid any fruit jellies.

YIELD: 4 SERVINGS

BAKED PEARS

The warmth of tart pears topped with a nutty crumble and a creaminess of yogurt—just wow! Like a sweet blanket hugging your tastebuds (especially on a chilly night), this decadent recipe is truly elegant but also simple enough to whip up on the spot without hours of labor or advance planning. Be sure to source the freshest pears available to you, and don't be shy with the cannabis-infused honey.

+ TARGET DOSE:

Your preferred dose (using Cannabis-Infused Honey, page 50)

+ EQUIPMENT:

9-by-13-inch baking dish

Parchment paper

+ INGREDIENTS:

For the pears:

2 pears cut in half lengthwise

2 tablespoons browned butter

Pinch nutmeg

¼ teaspoon vanilla extract

⅛ teaspoon ginger

For the crumble:

¼ cup vanilla wafers, or any simple vanilla butter–based cookie of your choice, crushed

2 tablespoons pistachios, chopped

2 tablespoons pecans, chopped

2 tablespoons sliced almonds

½ teaspoon cinnamon

2 tablespoons honey (noninfused)

1 tablespoon cornstarch

2 tablespoons melted butter

Pinch of salt

Almond yogurt or whipped mascarpone cheese

Crushed pistachios, for garnish

Drizzle of Cannabis-Infused Honey at your preferred dose (page 50)

1. Preheat the oven to 375°F (190°C).
2. In a small bowl, mix together the crushed cookies, pistachios, pecans, almonds, cinnamon, honey, cornstarch, melted butter, and salt until sticky and clumpy. Set aside.
3. In another small bowl, whisk in the browned butter, nutmeg, vanilla extract, and ginger.
4. Place the pears, cut side up, in a baking dish; brush the brown butter mixture all over the pears.
5. Bake the pears for about 20 minutes.
6. Brush on another layer of the brown butter mixture, and top with the crumble.
7. Bake for another 10 to 15 minutes until the pears are fork tender and the crumble is crispy and brown.
8. Smear a generous layer of almond yogurt on a dessert plate, drizzle with your desired amount of Cannabis-Infused Honey, and sprinkle crushed pistachios on top.
9. Place the baked pears on top of the almond yogurt, and enjoy!

> *Tip!* To save time, skip step 2 completely; you can always use a nutty granola as a topping. The almond yogurt really accentuates the flavors of this dish, but you can also swap it for regular yogurt, whipped cream, mascarpone cheese, or even a scoop of ice cream.

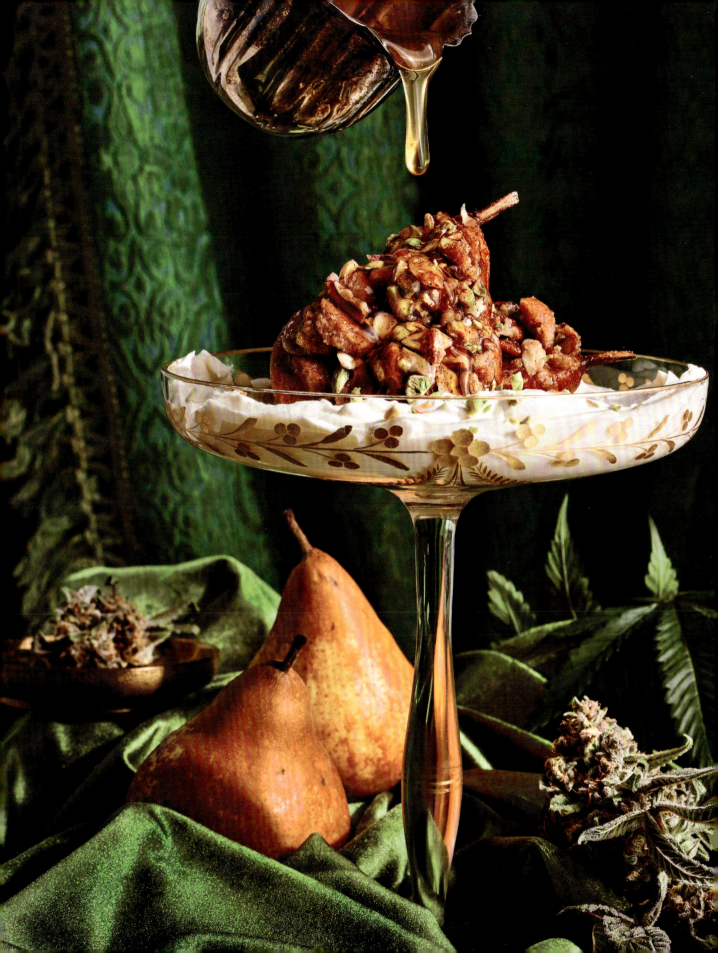

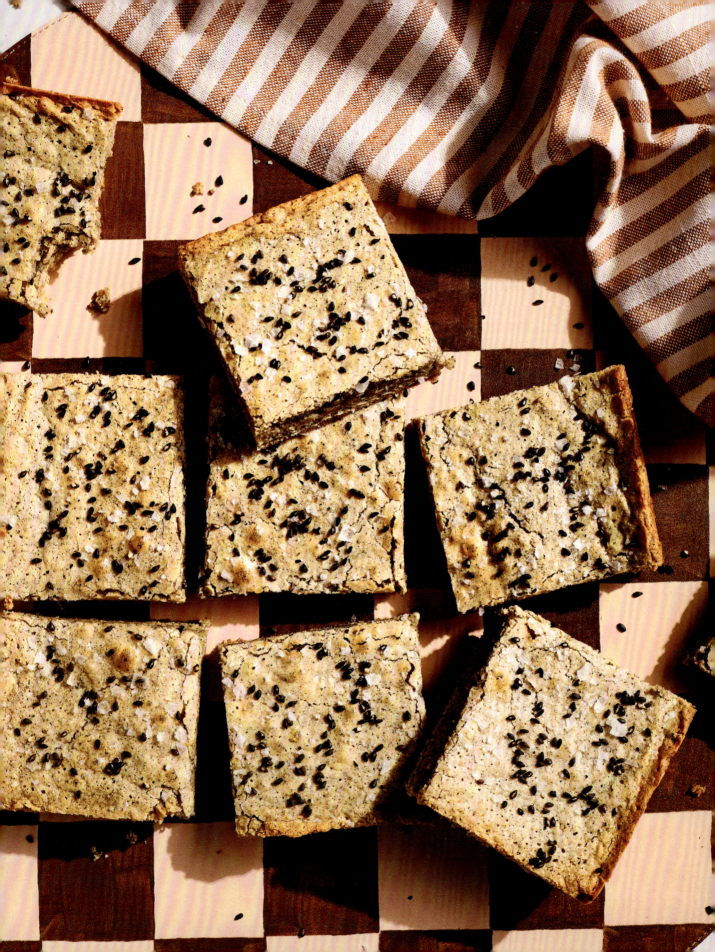

YIELD: 9 TO 12 SQUARES

BLACK SESAME BLONDIE

Pot brownies—the most popular edible of all the edibles! But let's be honest, it's been done and done again. This black sesame blondie recipe is our take on the popular stoner classic, but our dish is both sweet and savory, with a unique nutty flavor. If you're new to blondies, they're basically a brownie but without the chocolate, acting as a perfect base to incorporate a variety of add-ins and flavors. Be sure to sprinkle with Maldon salt and more black sesame for an extra boost of flavor! This recipe is the perfect way to incorporate cannabis without it tasting too much like weed.

+ TARGET DOSE:

Your preferred dose (using Cannabis-Infused Powdered Sugar, page 51)

+ EQUIPMENT:

8-by-8-inch square baking pan
Measuring cups
Measuring spoons
Stand mixer or handheld mixer

+ INGREDIENTS:

1 cup light brown sugar, packed
2 eggs, at room temperature
¼ cup granulated sugar
1 teaspoon vanilla extract
1 teaspoon almond extract
½ teaspoon salt
½ cup browned butter
½ cup condensed milk
½ cup toasted black sesame seeds, ground
1 cup all-purpose flour
½ teaspoon baking powder
Maldon salt and extra black sesame, for sprinkling
Cannabis-Infused Powdered Sugar, sifted, at your preferred dosage (page 51)

1. Preheat the oven to 350°F (176°C).
2. Grease an 8-by-8-inch baking pan.
3. In a large mixing bowl, combine the brown sugar, eggs, granulated sugar, vanilla extract, almond extract, and salt. Mix until thick and fluffy.
4. In a separate medium-size bowl, mix together the browned butter, condensed milk, and black sesame seed powder until mixed through. Add to the egg mixture a little at a time.
5. Gradually sift the flour and baking powder into the wet batter, and gently fold with a silicone spatula.
6. Pour the mixture into the greased baking pan, and let bake for about 20 minutes.
7. Remove the blondies from the oven. Give the pan a good slam, to remove any excess air and achieve the texture of a brownie or blondie.
8. Sprinkle some extra black sesame seeds and Maldon salt on top.
9. Return the blondies to the oven for another 15 minutes or until a toothpick comes out clean.
10. When cool, sift the Cannabis-Infused Powdered Sugar on top. Cut, and enjoy!

Tip! If you can't find toasted black sesame seeds in a powdered form, you can grind them with a spice grinder. To make the browned butter, just heat butter on the stove on high, mixing constantly until you have a caramel brown color. See page 51 on how to turn your infused sugar into powdered sugar.

YIELD: 12 MINI CHEESECAKES

MINI BLUEBERRY CHEESECAKE BITES

Perfect for parties or entertaining, these Mini Blueberry Cheesecake Bites are only half-baked, so they come together easily and are just so dang cute! Incorporating all the classic cheesecake flavors with a pop of blueberry, these bite-size treats are simple to create and are a guaranteed crowd-pleaser. The infused coconut whipped cream on top gives you an easily controlled dosage for individual servings. Just be sure to have some mini cupcake liners at home to bake these into the right shape.

+ TARGET DOSE:

6 mg THC | <1 mg CBD per serving (using Cannabis-Infused Coconut Cream, page 63)

+ EQUIPMENT:

Mini cupcake liners with foil

+ INGREDIENTS:

¼ cup speculoos cookie or graham cracker cookie crumbs

¼ cup whole pecans

2 tablespoons butter

Pinch of salt

1 cup frozen blueberries

¼ cup water

¼ cup granulated sugar

1 cup cream cheese, softened at room temperature

⅓ cup granulated sugar

½ cup Cannabis-Infused Coconut Cream (page 63)

1 cup heavy whipping cream

3 cups powdered sugar

1. Preheat the oven to 350°F (176°C).
2. Combine the speculoos and pecans in a food processor, and pulse until they are small crumbs. Add the butter and a pinch of salt. Pulse until well combined.
3. Carefully press a spoonful of the crumble mixture into the cupcake liners, and gently press to shape the bottoms. Repeat until you've used all the crumbly mixture.
4. Place in the oven for about 7 minutes. Let cool.
5. In a saucepan on medium heat, add the blueberries, water, and sugar. Bring to a boil; then lower heat to a simmer for another 15 minutes, stirring occasionally.
6. Blend the blueberry purée; strain through a fine-mesh sieve, using a spoon to push the contents through. Discard the rest.
7. When the blueberry purée has completely cooled, use a handheld mixer to whip it thoroughly with the cream cheese and sugar. Add the infused coconut cream, and whip until completely smooth.
8. Spoon the blueberry cream cheese on top of the speculoos crust in your cupcake liners. Spread it evenly, making sure it is distributed to all the edges of the cupcake liner.
9. Place the mini cheesecakes in the fridge to set for at least 6 hours.
10. In a large mixing bowl, using a hand mixer, whip the heavy cream and powdered sugar until stiff peaks form.
11. Once set, remove the cheesecakes from the fridge. Top with the whipped cream, and then enjoy!

YIELD: 8 SERVINGS (ABOUT 18 CASHEWS PER SERVING)

HONEY FURIKAKE CASHEWS

Crunchy, sweet, and savory, these microdosed nuts are the perfect pop-into-your-mouth snack! If you're looking for an easy-to-make edible, this recipe can be prepared in 15 minutes or less. All you need are whole cashews, sesame seeds, honey, cannabis-infused butter, plus a few other tasty items to create at home. These treats are impossible to only have one, especially when binge-watching your favorite show, so be mindful of how many milligrams of cannabis you're consuming—it's easy to get carried away!

+ TARGET DOSE:

2 mg THC | 0 mg CBD per serving (using Cannabis-Infused Butter, page 48)

+ EQUIPMENT:

Sheet pan

Parchment paper

+ INGREDIENTS:

8 ounces whole cashews

2 tablespoons honey

2 teaspoons Cannabis-Infused Butter (page 48)

2 tablespoons raw sesame seeds

½ teaspoon salt

2 tablespoons furikake

1. Preheat the oven to 200°F (93°C).
2. In a mixing bowl, combine the cashews, honey, Cannabis-Infused Butter, and sesame seeds. Mix until the cashews are fully coated.
3. Spread the cashews evenly on a large sheet pan lined with parchment paper.
4. Place the sheet pan in the middle rack of the oven for 20 minutes.
5. Remove from the oven. Immediately sprinkle the salt and furikake over the cashews, and toss in the parchment paper.
6. Let cool, and enjoy!

> *Tip!* **Swap out almost any other whole nut for this recipe. Almonds and pecans work wonderfully with this mix, too!**

YIELD: 12 TO 18 COOKIES

JASMINE & CONDENSED MILK SANDWICH COOKIES

What isn't there to love about sandwich cookies? Two cookies in one, with a creamy, frosty filling holding it all together like a sweet group hug. There's something so delicious about condensed milk that we're absolutely obsessed with it, and the vanilla bean and floral jasmine truly shine together. The butter crumble of the cookies is the perfect texture to hold the soft, fluffy cannabis-infused cream together. This is truly one of the most memorable cookies you will ever have!

+ TARGET DOSE:

8 mg THC per serving (using Cannabis-Infused Butter, page 48)

+ EQUIPMENT:

Stand mixer with paddle
Silicone spatula
Rolling pin
Parchment paper
Saucepan
Cooling rack
Baking sheet
Measuring spoon
Measuring cups
2-inch cookie cutter
Piping bag

1. Combine the flour, baking powder, and salt in a medium bowl; set aside.
2. Using the paddle attachment on the mixer on medium speed, whip the sugar and butter until airy and light, about 5 minutes.
3. Add the egg and vanilla, and continue to mix, about 1 to 2 minutes.
4. Switch the mixer to low speed, and gradually add the flour mixture until everything starts coming together, about 2 to 3 minutes. Scrape down the sides with your silicone spatula as needed.
5. Remove the dough, and place onto a clean work surface. Knead until the dough comes together. Be careful not to overwork the dough.
6. Divide the dough evenly in half using a scale, and shape into 2 even disks. Wrap each disk separately in plastic wrap, making sure it is tight, with no air able to penetrate the dough.
7. Chill for 1 to 2 hours. The dough can last in the fridge up to 3 days before use.
8. Preheat the oven to 350°F (176°C).
9. Let the dough slightly soften at room temperature, about 10 to 15 minutes.
10. Remove the plastic wrap, and roll out the dough with a rolling pin between two sheets of parchment paper as evenly as possible. You'll want about ⅛-inch thickness in the dough. For an extra-even and level surface, you can gently press a large baking sheet on top of the dough. Remove the parchment paper.

* Recipe continued on page 83

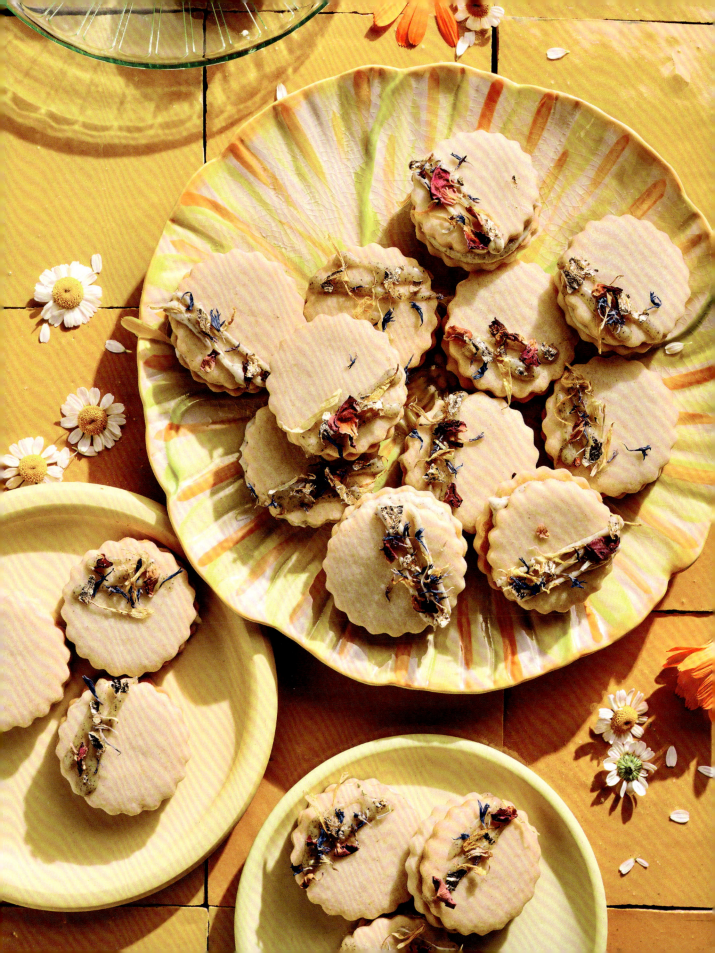

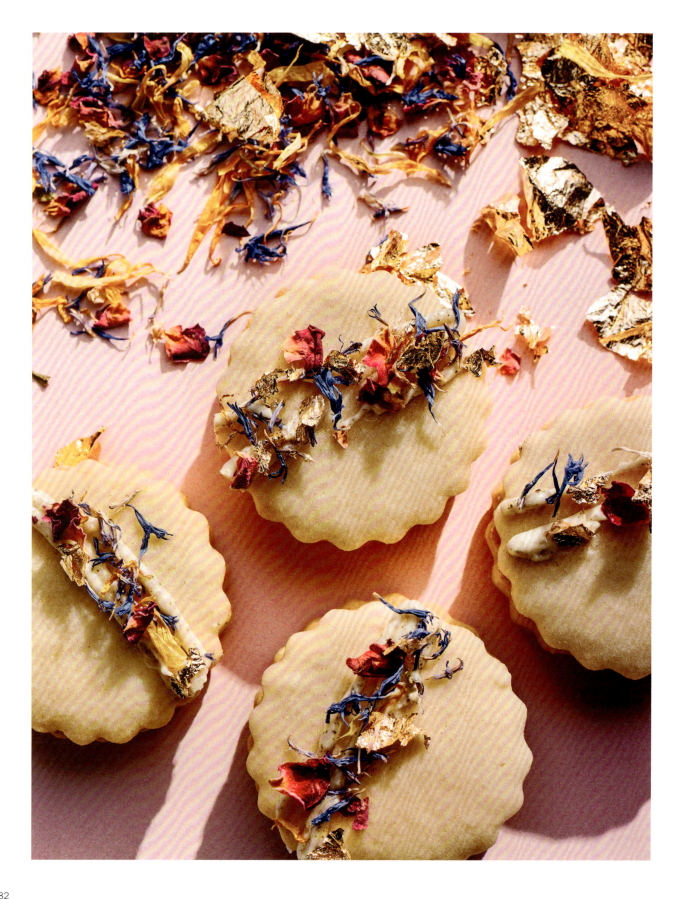

+ INGREDIENTS:

For the cookies:

1½ cups all-purpose flour, sifted

½ teaspoon baking powder

½ teaspoon salt

½ cup granulated sugar

½ cup butter, softened

1 small egg

½ teaspoon vanilla extract

For the filling:

One 14-ounce can condensed milk

¾ tablespoon jasmine tea leaves, powdered

½ vanilla bean, scraped

3 tablespoons cornstarch

¼ cup unsalted butter

¼ cup Cannabis-Infused Butter (page 48)

Additional powdered sugar, for desired sweetness (optional)

Pinch of salt

11. Using a 2-inch cookie cutter, cut 12 cookies from each sheet of dough. (We're using a fluted circle, but feel free to use whatever fun cookie cutters you have!) You should have 24 cookie circles.

12. Arrange the cookies on a parchment-lined baking sheet, spacing them apart. Place the baking sheet in the freezer for about 10 minutes to firm up the dough before baking.

13. Bake in the middle rack of the oven for 10 minutes, just until baked through but not browned.

14. Let the cookies rest for 2 to 3 minutes, and then transfer to a rack to finish cooling.

15. For the filling, heat the condensed milk, jasmine tea leaves, and vanilla bean. Simmer on low for about 3 minutes. Add the cornstarch, and heat for another 1 to 2 minutes. Remove from heat, and let cool completely.

16. In a large mixing bowl, add both the butter and the Cannabis-Infused Butter, and whip until smooth. Add the condensed milk mixture, and mix until well incorporated.

17. Gradually add powdered sugar 1 teaspoon at a time to achieve your desired sweetness and consistency for the filling.

18. Add the mixture to a piping bag.

19. Arrange 12 cookies upside down, and pipe about 2½ teaspoons of filling onto the middle of each cookie. Place the remaining 12 cookies on top of the filling to make a sandwich cookie. Gently press the cookies together just until the filing spreads toward the edges.

20. Decorate, and enjoy!

> *Tip!* Have fun decorating these however you want! This is our favorite part of the process. We used a little thinned-out filling to make a runny frosting and added gold flakes and dried edible flowers. You can keep it as simple or go as over the top as you want!

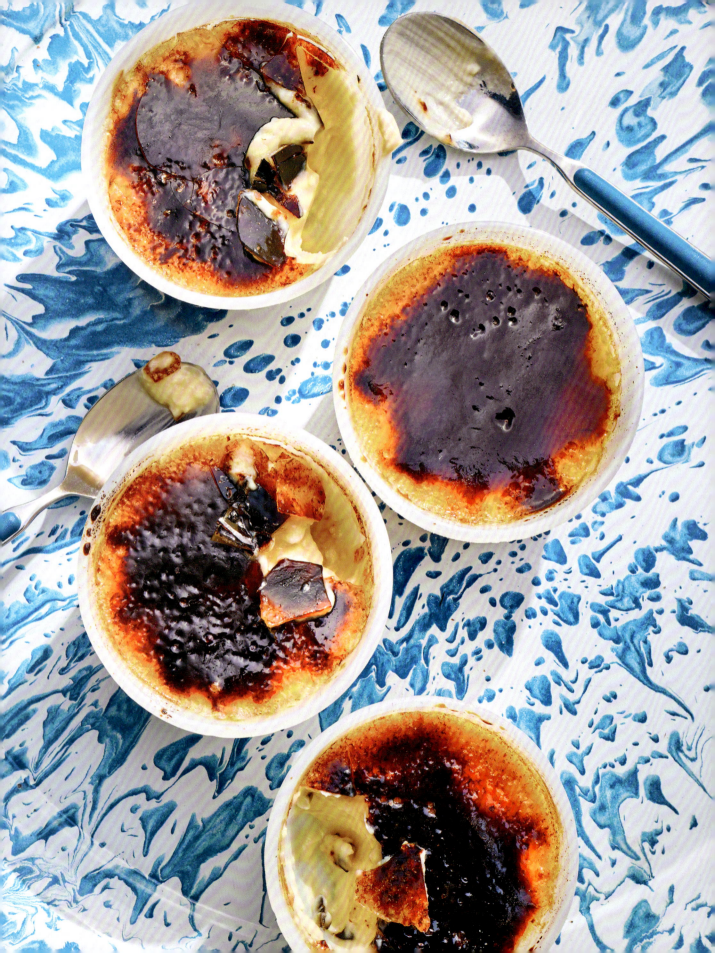

YIELD: 4 SERVINGS

MISO CRÈME BRÛLÉE

For a slightly salty, umami twist on a traditional classic, the miso in this crème brûlée adds a unique depth of flavor to this rich, silky, vanilla custard–based sweet treat—a truly fantastic combination of flavors! The satisfying-to-crack caramelized sugar crust is not only the signature of any crème brûlée, but also the perfect textural complement to the velvety smooth cream.

+ TARGET DOSE:

5 mg THC per serving (using Cannabis-Infused Sugar, page 51)

+ EQUIPMENT:

Culinary torch
Whisk
Saucepan
Mixing bowl
Measuring spoons
Measuring cups
Fine-mesh sieve
Four 6-ounce ramekins or ceramic cups

+ INGREDIENTS:

1 teaspoon white miso
½ teaspoon water
2 cups heavy cream
½ cup sugar
1 teaspoon Cannabis-Infused Sugar (page 51)
4 large egg yolks
1 teaspoon vanilla extract (or ½ a vanilla bean, scraped)
¼ cup sugar for torching

Tip! **Make sure you buy a white miso without dashi (fish stock) added to it.**

1. Preheat the oven to 325°F (176°C).
2. In a small bowl, mix the white miso with ½ teaspoon water until it forms a runny paste. Shake the mixture through a small fine-mesh sieve to remove any tiny clumps so that your créme brûlée stays as smooth as possible. Set aside.
3. Combine the heavy cream, sugar, infused sugar, and miso paste in a saucepan over low to medium heat, stirring occasionally, until the sugar has dissolved. Remove from heat. (Do not bring to a boil; low and slow is key.)
4. In a medium mixing bowl, whisk egg yolks and vanilla until thoroughly combined.
5. Slowly pour ¼ of the hot cream into the egg mix, making sure to continuously whisk so the eggs do not cook or separate. Continue with the rest of the mixture in small increments so the eggs do not cook and are slowly brought to temperature with the cream. (*Tip:* This technique is called tempering.)
6. Strain the mixture through a fine-mesh sieve. Don't skip this process; it is important to create that silky, velvety texture.
7. Pour the mixture into your ramekins and place them into a baking dish filled with hot water that reaches to just about halfway up the side of the ramekin.
8. Bake at 325°F (162°C) for about 30 minutes, or until the custard is set but still jiggly in the center.
9. Remove the ramekins from the oven and water bath, letting them cool to room temperature.
10. Once cool, cover the top of the ramekins with plastic wrap and let them completely chill in the fridge for at least 3 hours (or overnight).
11. When you are ready to enjoy, remove the plastic wrap and sprinkle enough sugar to evenly cover the entire top of the custard (about 1 tablespoon for each crème brûlée).
12. Using your culinary torch, melt the sugar until it browns and liquifies, moving over the surface in small but quick increments. When it's cooled, the liquified sugar will harden and form a crispy, caramelized layer on top.

YIELD: 12 TO 15 SERVINGS

STRAWBERRY MATCHA SHORTCAKE CUPS

Strawberry shortcake was an all-time favorite growing up. A deli down the street sold them in premade cups or in ice cream form, and they were such a treat. A little slice of heaven, this recipe adds a grown-up, sophisticated spin with matcha cream that perfectly compliments not only the strawberries, but also the terpenes in the cannabis. Because these are individual servings in jars, you can make them ahead of time and keep them in the fridge until you are ready to serve.

+ TARGET DOSE:

4 to 5 mg THC per serving (using Cannabis-Infused Powdered Sugar, page 51)

+ EQUIPMENT:

Stand mixer or handheld mixer

+ INGREDIENTS:

¾ cup unsalted butter, softened

1½ cups granulated sugar

4 large eggs

1½ teaspoons vanilla extract

2 cups all-purpose flour, sifted

½ teaspoon baking soda

½ teaspoon baking powder

½ teaspoon salt

1 cup sour cream, divided

3 cups heavy cream

¾ cup powdered sugar

1 tablespoon Cannabis-Infused Powdered Sugar (page 51)

½ teaspoon vanilla extract

2 tablespoons powdered matcha

2 pounds strawberries, diced

3 tablespoons granulated sugar

Pinch of salt

1. Preheat the oven to 350°F (176°C).
2. In a stand mixer with a paddle attachment, whip together the butter and sugar until smooth and fluffy.
3. Add the eggs, one by one, on medium speed; then add the vanilla.
4. In a separate, medium-size bowl, mix together the flour, baking soda, baking powder, and salt.
5. Add half the flour mix to the butter and sugar, mixing until just combined. Add half the sour cream until just combined. Repeat, and be careful not to overmix.
6. Grease and flour the baking sheet, or line with parchment paper. Pour the batter onto the baking sheet, and spread evenly.
7. Bake for about 20 minutes on the middle rack or until a toothpick comes out clean. Cool, and set aside.
8. In a large mixing bowl, whip the heavy cream until thickened.
9. Add the infused and regular powdered sugar, vanilla, and matcha to the whipped cream, just until stiff peaks form. Be careful not to overwhip the cream.
10. In a mixing bowl, toss together the strawberries with the sugar. Set aside.
11. Cut 24 small cake rounds, the same diameter as the cups you are using to assemble. We used a 2-inch circle cookie cutter and 2-inch-wide cups. You'll need 2 cut rounds of cake per 1 shortcake cup.
12. To assemble, place 2 cake rounds at the bottom layer of your dessert cup, add a layer of strawberries, and then add a layer of matcha cream. Repeat for each cup.
13. Garnish with another strawberry and a dust of powdered matcha, and enjoy!

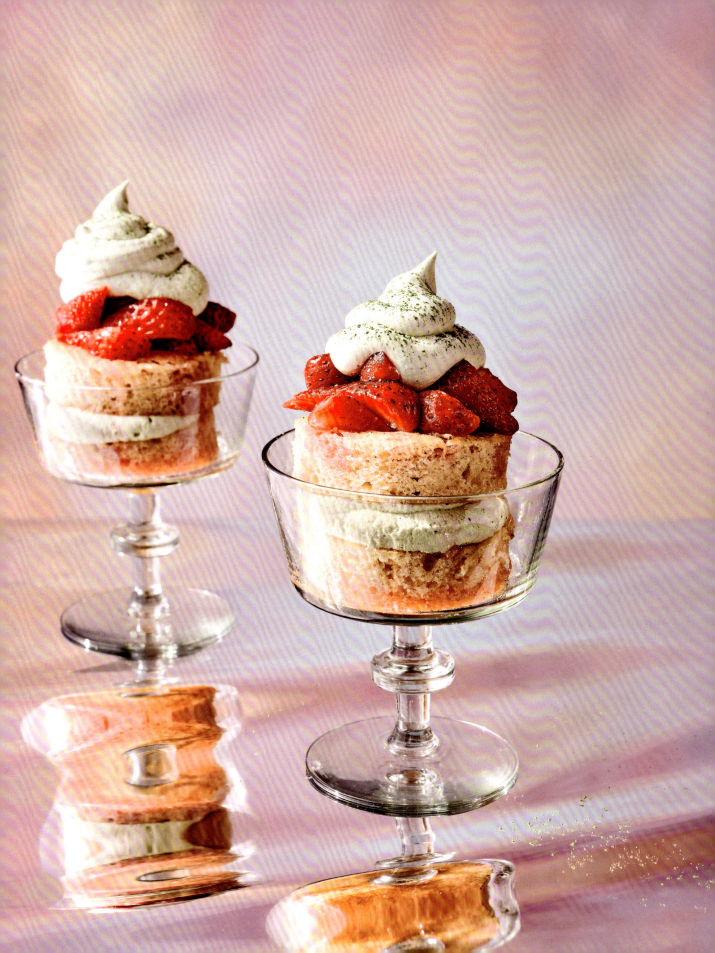

BAKED SAVORY

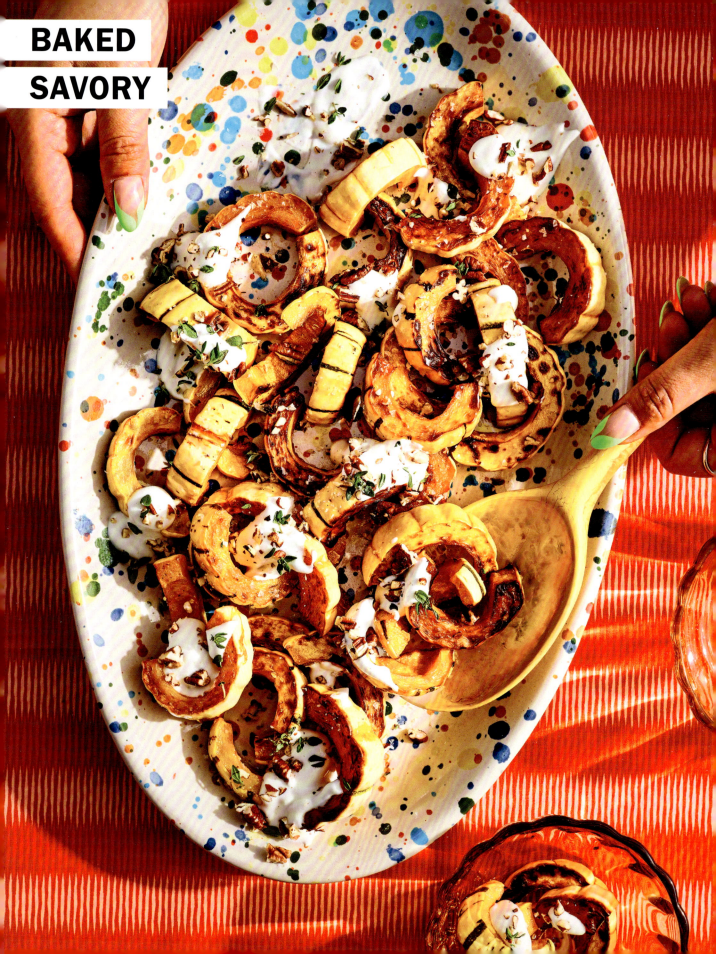

YIELD: 2 TO 4 SERVINGS

DELICATA SQUASH WITH GOAT CHEESE & HONEY

In this dish, a humble squash is transformed into something surprisingly elegant and flavorful! Pairing the tender, earthy squash with the creamy goat cheese and sweet honey results in a combination of flavors and textures that work harmoniously together. It's a simple side dish to accompany any cozy dinner at home, as well as a perfect dish to share with family and friends during the holidays. The honey is the infused element here and one of the final garnishes, so feel free to dose to your preference.

+ TARGET DOSE:

Your preferred dose (using Cannabis-Infused Honey, page 50)

+ EQUIPMENT:

Sheet pan
Measuring spoon
Parchment paper

+ INGREDIENTS:

1 delicata squash
2 tablespoons olive oil
¼ teaspoon salt
Pinch of black pepper
4 ounces goat cheese
½ teaspoon olive oil
1 teaspoon water
Pinch of salt
Drizzle of Cannabis-Infused Honey at your preferred dose (page 50)
Toasted pecans and thyme, for garnish (optional)

1. Preheat the oven to 375°F (191°C).
2. Cut the delicata squash in half, remove all the seeds, and then cut into 1-inch crescent moons.
3. Toss the squash with olive oil, salt, and pepper.
4. Spread the squash evenly on a sheet pan lined with parchment paper.
5. Roast the squash in the oven for about 10 to 15 minutes until the pieces are browned and fork tender. Then remove from the oven, and let cool.
6. Whip the goat cheese with ½ teaspoon of the olive oil and water until smooth.
7. Plate the squash, add dollops of goat cheese, drizzle with infused honey, and garnish with toasted pecans and thyme (optional). Enjoy!

YIELD: 8 PUFF PASTRIES

BULGOGI BBANG PUFF PASTRY

The word *bbang* in Korean means "bread," but it was also one of my favorite words to say growing up because it just sounds fun! Bulgogi (meaning "fire meat") is a well-known Korean BBQ meat that is thinly sliced and marinated. Most commonly made from beef, this flavorful protein is grilled on a barbecue or on a stovetop griddle, but for this recipe, we're wrapping it in a puff pastry. Stuffed into a pocket-size savory, buttery, flakey crust, you can never have enough of this delightful Bulgogi Bbang. We love a savory pastry, especially when it is infused with cannabis.

+ TARGET DOSE:

About 0.5 mg THC per 1 teaspoon of dipping sauce (using Cannabis-Infused Chili Oil, page 47, and Cannabis-Infused Honey, page 50)

+ EQUIPMENT:

Mixing bowl
Saucepan
Baking sheet
Measuring spoons
Measuring cups
Silicone brush

+ INGREDIENTS:

For the puff pastry:

1 tablespoon vegetable oil
1 cup chopped onions
1 cup mushrooms, diced
¼ cup soy sauce
¼ cup brown sugar
1 tablespoon rice wine vinegar
1 tablespoon grated ginger
1 tablespoon minced garlic
1½ tablespoons sesame oil
½ teaspoon black pepper
1 pound lean grass-fed ground beef
½ cup chopped chives
1 egg
1 tablespoon flour
¼ cup cooked and chopped sweet potato noodles
14 ounces puff pastry, thawed
1 egg beaten, for egg wash
2 tablespoons sesame seeds

For the dipping sauce:

½ cup sour cream
½ tablespoon chipotle powder
¼ teaspoon black pepper
¼ teaspoon lime juice
Pinch of salt
2 tablespoons freshly chopped chives
1 tablespoon Cannabis-Infused Chili Oil (12 mg) (page 47)
1 teaspoon Cannabis-Infused Honey (4 mg) (page 50)

1. Preheat the oven to 400°F (204°C).
2. In a saucepan, cook the chopped onions and mushrooms with vegetable oil on medium heat until tender and lightly browned. Let cool completely.
3. In a large mixing bowl, combine the soy sauce, brown sugar, vinegar, ginger, garlic, sesame oil, and black pepper. Whisk together to make the marinade.
4. Add the beef, cooked vegetables, chives, egg, flour, and cooked sweet potato noodles to the marinade.
5. Using gloves, thoroughly combine everything by hand so it's completely mixed.
6. Lay out the puff pastry. Cut 1 sheet into 8 even pieces. Repeat on the second sheet so you have 16 pieces of puff pastry to work with.
7. Using a spring-loaded ice cream or cookie scoop, add 1 scoop of the bulgogi meat mixture to the middle of each of the 8 puff pastry squares.
8. Brush pastry edges with egg wash.
9. Place the other 8 pieces of puff pastry on top of the meat mixture, gently pressing down to make them more uniform. Using a fork, press down all the edges to seal.
10. Brush the egg wash the top of the pastry, and sprinkle with sesame seeds.
11. Cut 3 tiny slits at the top of each pastry to allow steam to escape.
12. Lay out the pastries on a baking sheet lined with parchment paper. Bake for 20 to 25 minutes or until the pastries are golden brown on top.
13. For the dipping sauce, combine all the sauce ingredients in a small bowl, and mix together until thoroughly incorporated.

> **Tip!** **Cook a small spoonful of the meat in a pan. Taste to make sure the seasoning is to your liking, and add salt or more soy sauce as needed before you stuff all the pastries. These taste amazing on their own, but if you want to make a dipping sauce for them, a spicy aioli works great.**

YIELD: 4 TO 6 SERVINGS

CHEESY KIMCHI & TOMATO DIP

Mmmm, an ooey, gooey, cheesy kimchi and tomato dip—we are already drooling! This explosive savory dip is one of the showstoppers featured in this book. Your guests will continuously ask for this fan-favorite recipe, so be sure to bookmark this page! This mouth-watering appetizer is best served with crispy rice chips (see page 94), but any chip will do. We hope you enjoy this unforgettable party in your mouth, perfect for any gathering or group occasion.

+ TARGET DOSE:

0.25 mg THC per tablespoon of dip (using Cannabis-Infused Sesame Oil, page 44)

+ EQUIPMENT:

8-inch cast iron or oven-safe skillet

Baking sheet lined with foil

Measuring spoons

Measuring cups

+ INGREDIENTS:

10 ounces cherry or sungold tomatoes

2 tablespoons red wine vinegar or apple cider vinegar

½ teaspoon olive oil

1 tablespoon sugar

½ teaspoon thyme

¼ cup unsalted butter

1½ cups chopped kimchi

¾ cup diced sweet onions

¼ cup dashi stock (any stock is fine, but dashi works best)

1 teaspoon fish sauce

¼ teaspoon black pepper

2 tablespoons kimchi juice, saved from the jar

½ tablespoon gochujang

1 tablespoon sugar

¼ cup crème fraîche or sour cream

¼ cup cream cheese

½ cup pepper jack cheese, divided

2 tablespoon thinly sliced scallions

½ tablespoon Cannabis-Infused Sesame Oil (page 44)

More scallions and toasted sesame seeds for garnishing

* Recipe continued on page 94

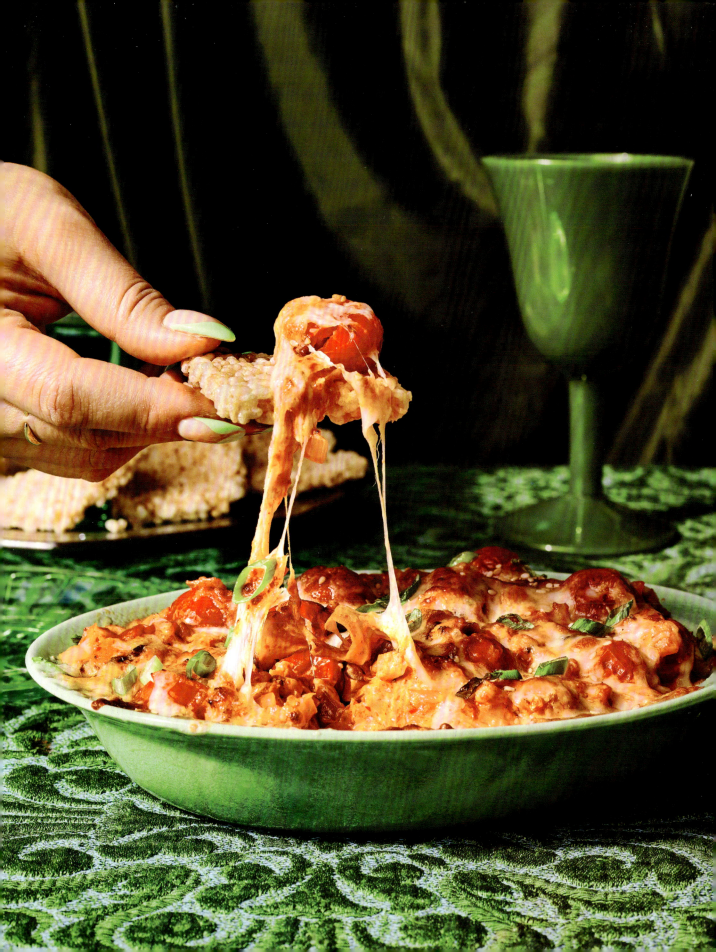

1. Preheat the oven to 450°F (232°C) with a foil-lined baking sheet inside.
2. Toss the tomatoes in the vinegar, olive oil, and sugar, and spread them out on your preheated baking sheet. Bake in the oven for about 5 to 7 minutes until the tomatoes have shrunk in size and caramelized and some moisture has cooked off.
3. Remove the tomatoes from the oven, add the thyme, and set aside.
4. In a skillet on low to medium heat, add the butter, kimchi, and onions. Sauté for about 5 minutes, stirring occasionally, until you get a darker red, jamlike texture.
5. Add the stock, fish sauce, pepper, kimchi juice, gochujang, and sugar to the mixture. Cook on medium-high heat, stirring often, until 75 percent of the moisture is gone.
6. Turn off the heat, but while the pan is still hot, add in the crème fraîche, the cream cheese, and half the pepper jack to the kimchi mixture. Stir until completely incorporated.
7. Gently fold in the blistered tomatoes and scallions.
8. Preheat the oven to 400°F (204°C).
9. Top the mixture with the other half of the pepper jack cheese.
10. Pop in the oven for about 12 minutes until everything is bubbling.
11. Top with 1 tablespoon Cannabis-Infused Sesame Oil, extra scallions, and toasted sesame seeds, and serve with your favorite rice cracker.

> *Tip!* **Poking a slit in each cherry tomato will ensure that the skin won't burst open.**
>
> *Tip!* **Our favorite rice crackers are ones you puff up fresh at home. Taking the extra time to fresh-fry these crispy rice chips is worth the effort, but any chip (wonton, tortilla, pita) will work with this dip.**

YIELD: 4 INDIVIDUAL PIES

GOCHUJANG DUNGENESS CRAB POT PIE

Why have chicken pot pie when you can have crab pot pie? The sweet, tender meat of a fresh Dungeness crab is our preference, but you can use any fresh crab your local grocery store has in stock. Gochujang is a fermented Korean chili paste with a unique depth of flavor that makes this dish a truly decadent luxury wrapped in comfort and nostalgia. If the crab pot pie wasn't already over the top, that final brush of infused bacon fat, with its subtle savory and smokey flavor, really makes this dish a star!

+ TARGET DOSE:

2 mg THC per serving (using Cannabis-Infused Bacon Fat, page 49)

+ EQUIPMENT:

4 ramekins
Measuring spoons
Measuring cups
Silicone brush
Mixing bowls
Large skillet
Rolling pin

+ INGREDIENTS:

For the crust:

2½ cups all-purpose flour
1 teaspoon salt
1 teaspoon sugar
1 cup cold butter, cut into small cubes
½ cup ice water

For the filling:

½ cup butter, divided
¼ cup chopped onions
¼ cup chopped celery
¼ cup chopped carrots
½ cup white corn
½ cup diced crimini mushrooms
½ tablespoon minced garlic
¼ teaspoon black pepper
1 teaspoon grated ginger
¼ cup all-purpose flour
1 cup chicken or seafood stock
½ cup heavy cream
½ tablespoon gochujang
1 pound fresh crab meat
¼ teaspoon salt
¼ cup chopped chives
¼ teaspoon fresh parsley
1 teaspoon Cannabis-Infused Bacon Fat (page 49)
1 egg beaten (for egg wash)

Recipe continued on page 97

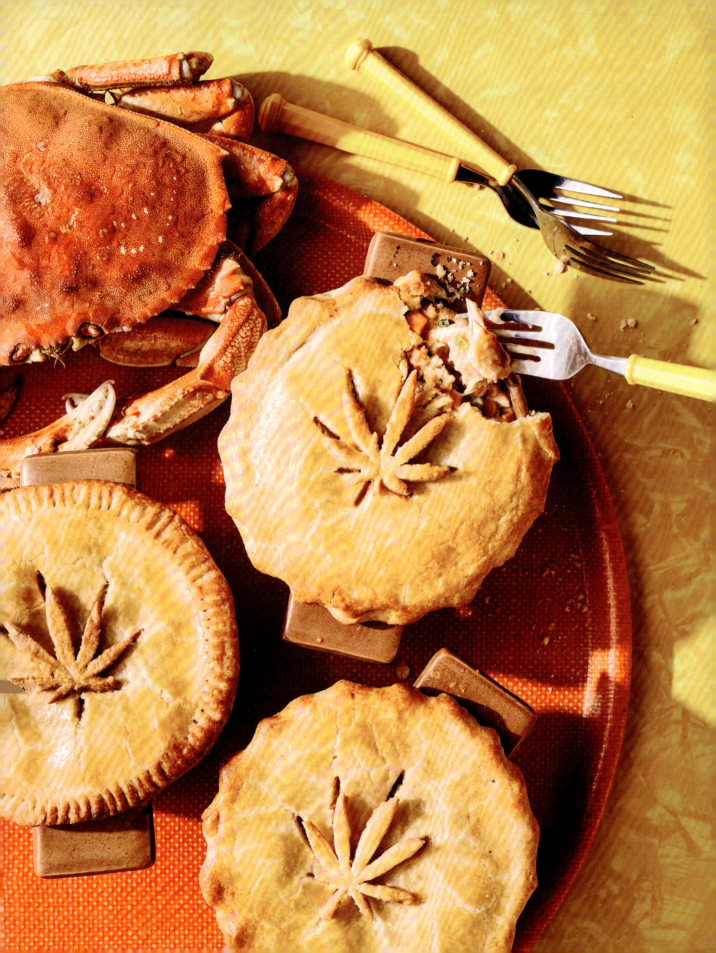

To make the crust:

1. Combine the flour, salt, sugar, and cubed butter in a large mixing bowl. Using your fingers, work the butter into the flour mixture until it's crumbly and everything is somewhat clumped together.
2. Gradually add in a small amount of ice water at time, mixing with a fork until the dough comes together. Form the dough into a ball or mound. Divide it into two equal pieces, flattening the dough into circles; wrap in plastic wrap. Put the dough in the fridge for 1 hour.
3. Preheat the oven to 375°F (190°C).

To make the filling:

1. Melt half the butter in a large skillet on medium heat, and add the chopped onions, celery, carrots, corn, and mushrooms. Sauté until tender. Add the garlic, black pepper, and ginger. Cook for 1 more minute. Transfer to a bowl, and set aside.
2. In the same skillet, add the rest of the butter on medium heat, and whisk in the flour until smooth.
3. Gradually add the chicken stock and heavy cream, constantly whisking until smooth and thick. Add the gochujang until it is dissolved and thoroughly mixed in.
4. Reintroduce the vegetables from step 4 into the pot of creamy goodness, and gently add the crab and the salt while folding everything together.
5. Turn off the heat, and mix in the fresh chives and parsley. Let cool to room temperature.
6. Using a rolling pin, roll out the chilled dough on a floured surface to about ⅛-inch thickness. Divide the dough into 4 equal parts. Repeat with the remaining dough.
7. Press and mold the dough carefully into four 6-inch pie dishes or ramekins. Cut off any excess dough.
8. Spoon the creamy crab-and-veggie filling into the pie dishes, filling each to the top.
9. Top each ramekin with the remaining 4 pieces of dough, cut off the excess around the rim, and use a fork or knife to pinch the edges of the top dough down.
10. Cut small slits at the top of each pie to allow steam to escape while cooking. Brush the entire top with the egg wash.
11. Bake for 45 to 50 minutes or until golden brown and bubbling hot.
12. Right before you pull out the pies, turn off the oven and brush each pie top with ¼ teaspoon of Cannabis-Infused Bacon Fat. Leave the pies in the oven with the fan on for about 2 minutes.
13. Remove the pies from the oven. Let cool before eating.

YIELD: 6 SERVINGS

STEAMED EGG + SHIITAKE + CHILI OIL

Delicious cloudlike whipped eggs steamed to custardy perfection make up this delicious dish. The toppings for this dreamy recipe can vary, depending on your preferences and your mood—everything from crab, to roasted kimchi, to just chili oil will work perfectly. However, the creaminess of the shiitake with the eggs and a kick of that infused chili oil is our favorite way to enjoy these pillowy soft eggs.

+ TARGET DOSE:

Your preferred dose (using Cannabis-Infused Chili Oil, page 47)

+ EQUIPMENT:

Pot with steamer insert
Foil
Tempered ceramic bowl
Whisk
Fine-mesh strainer
6 small teacups or ramekins
Mixing bowl
Measuring spoons
Measuring cups
Cake tester or toothpick

+ INGREDIENTS:

8 large eggs
4 cups dashi or any stock
1 tablespoon mirin
¼ tablespoon salt
2 tablespoons avocado oil
2 ounces sliced shiitake mushrooms
Pinch of salt
½ teaspoon sesame oil
Drizzle of Cannabis-Infused Chili Oil at your preferred dose (page 47)

1. Preheat the oven to 375°F (190°C).
2. Crack 6 large eggs into a medium mixing bowl, and whisk with the dashi, mirin, and salt until thoroughly combined and an even consistency.
3. Pour the mixture through a fine-mesh sieve. Then pour the refined mixture into 6 small teacups or ramekins. Cover each ramekin tightly with a piece of foil.
4. Bring a pot of water with a flat steamer to a boil, and then bring the heat to medium-low.
5. Gently place the ramekins in the steamer, and cover with a lid for about 20 to 30 minutes. Remove one ramekin from the steamer, lift the foil covering, and make sure it is fully set but still jiggly. Puncture with a cake tester or toothpick: If the water is running clear and not cloudy, it's ready.
6. Remove the egg custards, and set aside (with the foil still on).
7. In a small pan on medium heat, add 3 tablespoons avocado oil and the shiitake mushrooms. Cover with a lid. Stir the mushrooms occasionally until most of the excess moisture has cooked off and they have some color.
8. Remove the mushrooms from heat, and add a pinch of salt and a drizzle of sesame oil.
9. Remove the foil from the egg custards, top with the sautéed shiitake mushrooms, and add a generous drizzle of the Cannabis-Infused Chili Oil.

Tip! Make sure the water isn't boiling too much and doesn't get too hot. You want a gentle steam for the egg custards, or else the eggs will soufflé or steam over.

YIELD: 8 SERVINGS

JALAPEÑO CHIVE CORNBREAD

Cornbread is a simple and delicious addition to any meal. Made with cornmeal, a dash of honey, chopped green onions, diced jalapeños, and other tasty ingredients, this cornbread recipe is deliciously dense but with a light, fluffy crumble. If you're a cornbread lover, you're going to get down on this sweet and savory version of a beloved classic—with a little kick!

+ TARGET DOSE:

Your preferred dose (using Cannabis-Infused Butter, page 48, or Cannabis-Infused Honey, page 50)

+ EQUIPMENT:

Greased 8-inch baking pan or cast-iron pan (if you like crispier edges)

2 large mixing bowls

Whisk

Measuring cup

Parchment paper

+ INGREDIENTS:

1 cup cornmeal

1 cup all-purpose flour

1 tablespoon baking powder

½ tablespoon salt

¼ cup honey

2 large eggs

1 cup milk

½ cup melted butter, at room temperature

¼ cup chopped green onions

¼ cup diced jalapeños (add more if you want more spice)

Drizzle of your choice of Cannabis-Infused Butter (page 48) or Cannabis-Infused Honey (page 50)

1. Preheat the oven to 400°F (204°C).
2. Grease the pan with butter.
3. In a large mixing bowl, mix together all dry ingredients (cornmeal, flour, baking powder, salt).
4. In another large mixing bowl, whisk together all wet ingredients (honey, eggs, milk, butter).
5. Combine the wet ingredients into the dry ingredients, along with the green onions and jalapeños; stir until combined. Be careful not to overwork the batter. Pour the batter into a greased pan.
6. Bake for 20 to 25 minutes. When the cornbread is golden brown on top and a wooden toothpick comes out clean, remove it from the oven.
7. Allow the cornbread to cool slightly before slicing and serving.
8. Add a smear or drizzle of Cannabis-Infused Butter or Cannabis-Infused Honey, and enjoy!

YIELD: 3 SERVINGS

MISO GINGER GLAZED BLACK COD

This miso ginger glazed cod is a buttery, flakey whitefish broiled to perfection. Because of the fattiness, black cod is generally considered a beginner-friendly fish that is pretty much failsafe and won't dry out. Paired with the miso, ginger, and a quick broil (which adds a nice subtle smokey, caramelized flavor), this recipe not only comes together quickly but is a crowd favorite.

+ TARGET DOSE:

About 2 mg THC per serving (using Cannabis-Infused Sesame Oil, page 44)

+ EQUIPMENT:

Broiler
Sheet tray
Foil
Boning tweezers
Fish spatula

+ INGREDIENTS:

1 pound or 1 small filet black cod, portioned into 6-ounce filets

¼ cup mirin

¼ tablespoon grated ginger

2½ tablespoons white miso

1½ tablespoons brown sugar

¼ teaspoon black pepper

½ teaspoon soy sauce

1 teaspoon Cannabis-Infused Sesame Oil (page 44)

1. Portion your black cod filet into 3 even pieces (about 6 ounces each).
2. To make the glaze, in a small saucepan, combine the mirin, ginger, white miso, brown sugar, black pepper, and soy sauce. Bring the mixture to a simmer until the sugar and miso are well incorporated. Remove from heat, and whisk in the Cannabis-Infused Sesame Oil. Save 1½ tablespoons of this glaze, and set aside for brushing.
3. When the glaze has completely cooled, thoroughly coat the black cod filets, and place them in a sealable bag with the air pushed out. Make sure as much of the glaze is touching the cod as possible.
4. Store in the fridge for 2 hours.
5. When ready to cook, pull out the filets and set them on a foil-lined sheet pan with space in between each filet; let them rest to come to room temperature, about 15 minutes.
6. Set your oven to broil, and place your fish directly under the broiler for about 4 to 5 minutes. Check occasionally to make sure each filet is broiling evenly; you might need to rotate your pan to get an even broil.
7. When the fish is flakey and has a nice spotty char on top, remove from the broiler.
8. Use your deboning tweezers to carefully pull out any visible bones of the fish without breaking the flesh.
9. To the glaze that was set aside, whisk in 1 teaspoon Cannabis-Infused Sesame Oil. Using a silicone brush, brush each piece of fish with the glaze. Enjoy!

> *Tip!* **This cod works great with most sides, a bowl of rice, or vegetables. If you can't find black cod, Chilean sea bass is a great alternative.**

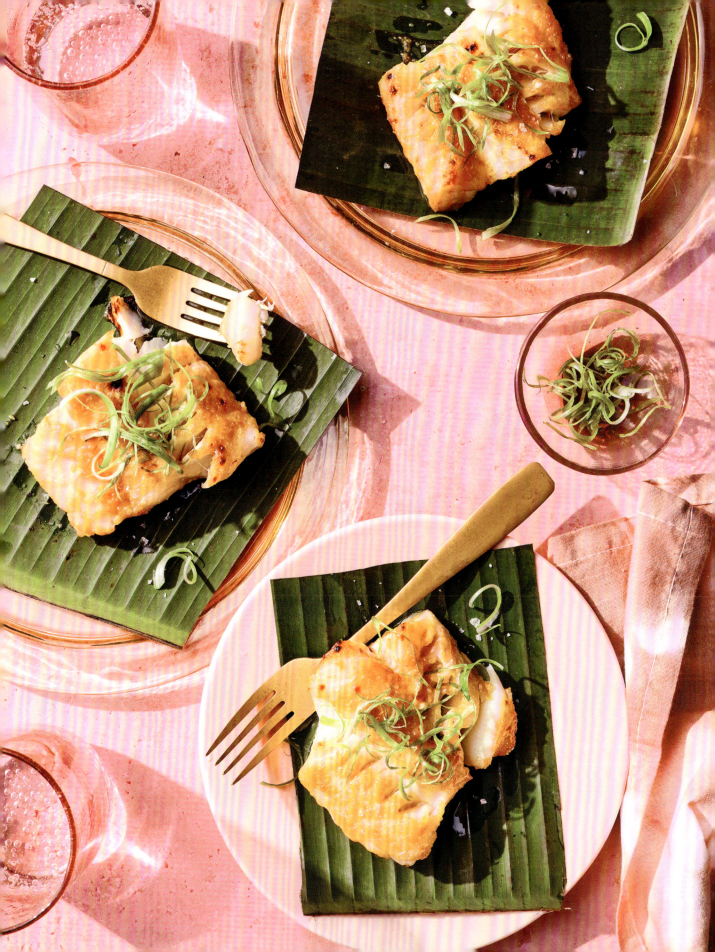

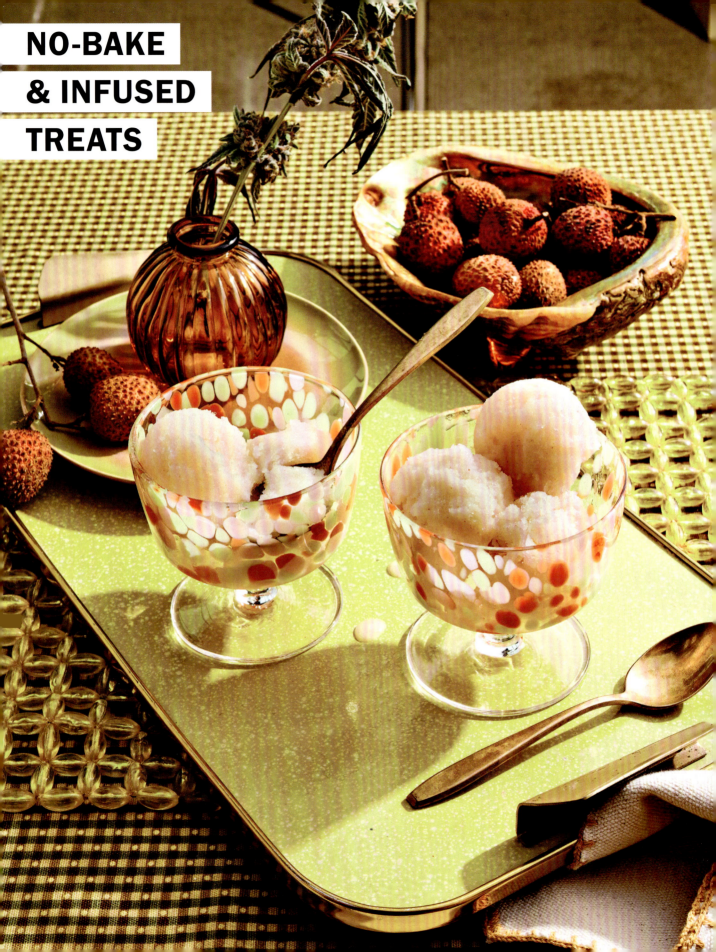

NO-BAKE & INFUSED TREATS

YIELD: 4 SERVINGS

LYCHEE SORBET

Lychee sorbet—we can't think of a more refreshing no-bake dessert. Not only is this sorbet a light palate cleanser, but its sweet, tangy, and floral ingredients blend together to create just the right flavors. When cooking or preparing drinks at home, try using lychee: It has one of the most unique and distinct fruit flavors. Incorporating it into a sorbet, this recipe is the perfect vehicle to showcase the lychee's delicate profile. Quick and simple, it's probably one of the easiest recipes in the entire book.

+ TARGET DOSE:

5 mg THC per serving (using Cannabis-Infused Sugar, page 51)

+ EQUIPMENT:

Blender

Shallow dish

+ INGREDIENTS:

One 20-ounce can peeled lychee in syrup

¼ cup lychee syrup (discard the rest)

1 tablespoon lime juice

1 teaspoon Cannabis-Infused Sugar (page 51)

¼ cup water

1. Strain the lychee from the syrup and freeze.
2. Blend the frozen lychee until smooth.
3. Transfer the mixture to a shallow dish, and freeze for 2 hours to set. Once it's fully frozen, let the sorbet sit out for 10 minutes before scooping, so it softens a bit.

> *Tip!* **You can always use fresh lychee as well, but make sure to peel and pit the fruit first.**

YIELD: 10 SERVINGS

DULCE DE LECHE PEACH TOAST

If you're a fan of peaches, you're going to love peaches mixed with dulce de leche. Yum—what a killer combination! Mixed together on top of fresh brioche bread, this simple yet stunning dish is easy to prepare at home. The buttery, airy crisp of the brioche creates a light but rich toast, making this recipe way too easy to overindulge in. Be sure to source the freshest peach you can find for the best flavor imaginable.

+ TARGET DOSE:

About 1.25 mg THC per tablespoon of whipped cream (using Cannabis-Infused Powdered Sugar, page 51)

+ EQUIPMENT:

Spatula

Pan

Saucepan

Rack

Bread knife

+ INGREDIENTS:

1 peach

¼ teaspoon maple syrup

1 tablespoon brown sugar

Pinch of salt

¼ teaspoon cinnamon

1 loaf brioche bread

1 tablespoon butter, softened (enough to spread on each side)

One 14-ounce can of dulce de leche

2 cups heavy whipping cream

2 teaspoons Cannabis-Infused Powdered Sugar (page 51)

1. Peel and pit the peach, and cut into thin, even slices.
2. In a medium saucepan, heat the maple syrup, brown sugar, salt, and cinnamon until fully combined. Add the peach slices. Gently swirl the pot in circles to coat the peaches evenly without damaging them too much from stirring. Set aside.
3. Cut the brioche loaf into 1¼-inch-thick slices, cutting off the crusts for a more even sear on each side. Butter all sides of the slices.
4. Preheat a large skillet on high heat, and add the brioche loaf, crisping every side until buttery and golden brown. Remove from heat, and place on a rack to cool.
5. Warm the dulce de leche either in a bowl in the microwave or in a saucepan on the stove, just until it is easily spreadable. Spread a thin layer on the brioche toast, face up. Add a layer of glazed peaches.
6. Whip the heavy cream and Cannabis-Infused Powdered Sugar until stiff peaks form; then add a couple scoops on top of the toast. Enjoy immediately.

Tip! **If you're lactose intolerant and can't have dairy, or if you can't find dulce de leche in stores, you can always substitute caramel or butterscotch.**

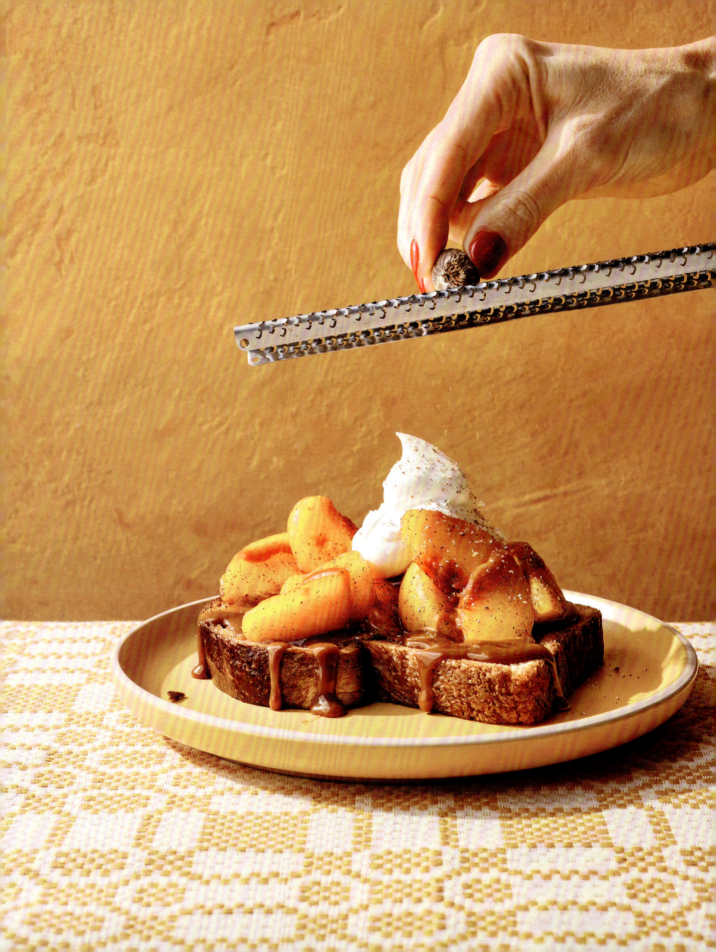

YIELD: 1 SERVING

CHOCO PIE MILKSHAKE

Choco Pie is a Korean cult-classic sweet treat, almost as famous as Oreos or Kit Kats! This scrumptious no-bake dessert is similar to a moon pie (two dense pieces of cake with marshmallows in the middle, covered in chocolate). Are you drooling yet? Made with cannabis-infused simple syrup, this easy-to-make recipe is perfect for those looking for a fast and efficient way to create enhanced sweets at home.

+ TARGET DOSE:

About 3.5 mg THC per serving (using Cannabis-Infused Simple Syrup, page 60)

+ EQUIPMENT:

Blender

+ INGREDIENTS:

2 Choco Pies (available at any Korean market)

2 cups vanilla ice cream

½ cup milk (oat, almond, or dairy milk recommended)

1 tablespoon cocoa powder

1 teaspoon vanilla extract

1 teaspoon Cannabis-Infused Simple Syrup (page 60)

1 tiny pinch of salt

1. Add all the ingredients to a blender. Blend until smooth.
2. Pour the mixture into a large glass, and enjoy immediately.

> *Tip!* **Childhood hack: Microwave the Choco Pie on a plate (remove the wrapper first) for about 15 to 20 seconds. You'll have a warm, s'more-like cake perfect for a late-night snack.**

YIELD: 12 TO 16 SERVINGS (DEPENDING ON THE SIZE OF SLICES)

MILK TEA–RAMISU

To introduce our take on the classic tiramisu, meet the Milk Tea–Ramisu! Swapping out the traditional espresso for a black milk tea is a yummy switch-up on this classic Italian dessert. Be sure to use a high-quality Earl Grey with hints of luscious bergamot to ensure that this version of tiramisu will be unforgettable. Great for entertaining, especially when expecting a group, this no-bake dessert can be made ahead of time and chilled until ready to serve.

+ TARGET DOSE:

125 mg THC for the entire cake, or 7.8 mg for 16 equal slices (using Cannabis-Infused Powdered Sugar, page 51)

+ EQUIPMENT:

9-by-13-inch baking dish
Whisk or hand mixer
Measuring spoons
Mixing bowls

+ INGREDIENTS:

40 grams (20 bags) Earl Grey tea
2 cups boiling water
1 cup condensed milk, divided
Pinch of salt
16 ounces mascarpone cheese
2 cups heavy cream
½ cup Cannabis-Infused Powdered Sugar (page 51)
½ teaspoon almond extract
½ teaspoon vanilla extract
30 ladyfinger cookies
Matcha or cocoa powder, for dusting

1. Steep 40 grams (20 bags) of Earl Grey tea in 2 cups of 90°F (32°C or boiling) water. Any hotter, and the tea can become bitter. Let steep for at least an hour.
2. When the tea is cool, strain all the tea leaves and add ¼ cup condensed milk to the tea. Set aside.
3. Mix the mascarpone cheese with 1 teaspoon condensed milk and a pinch of salt until creamy. Be sure to not overwork the cheese, or it will curdle.
4. Whip the heavy cream, powdered sugar, almond extract, and vanilla extract in a separate large mixing bowl until stiff peaks form.
5. Gently fold the whipped cream into the mascarpone, to keep it light and fluffy.
6. When the tea has completely cooled, dunk the ladyfingers in the tea, one at a time, and place them in a single layer at the bottom of a 9-by-13-inch baking dish.
7. Evenly smooth half the mascarpone cream mixture over the tea-soaked ladyfingers. Repeat steps 6 and 7 to create a second layer.
8. Cover, and pop into the fridge for at least 3 hours (or chill overnight).
9. Serve with a generous dusting of cocoa powder, or stay in the tea theme with a dusting of matcha powder.

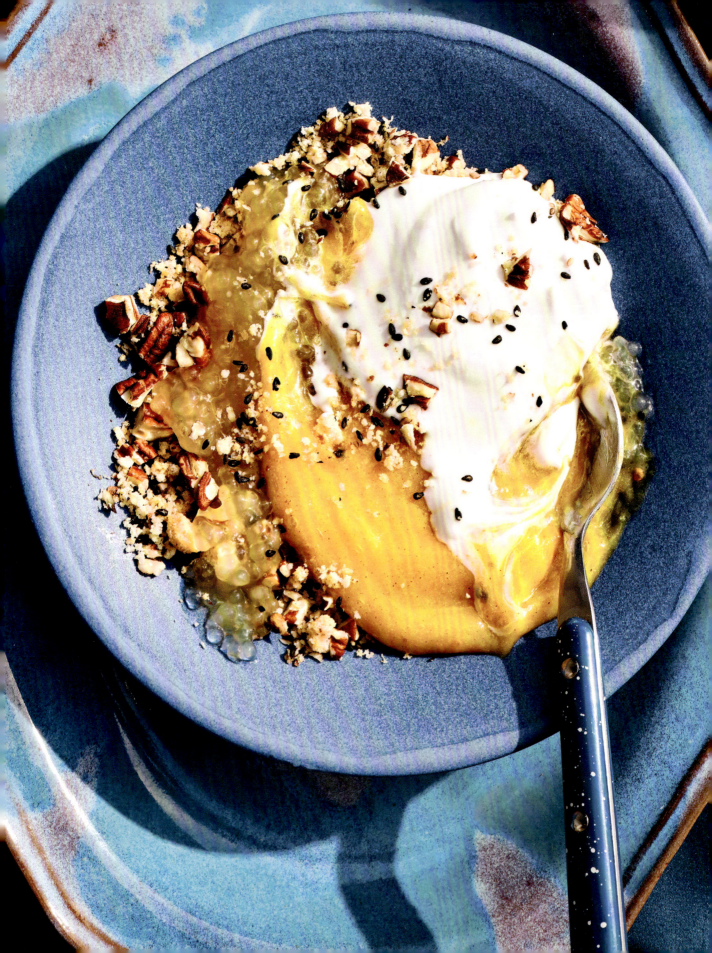

YIELD: ABOUT 12 DESSERT CUPS (4 TO 6 OUNCES EACH)

MANGO COCONUT TAPIOCA PUDDING

With so many different layers, flavors, and textures, this mango coconut tapioca pudding is the perfect spoonful of not-too-sweet airy, creamy goodness. When preparing this recipe at home, be sure to source fresh mangos, if possible, to enhance the flavor. If you have access to only canned or frozen mangoes, that works, too. Not only is this tasty tapioca visually stunning, but it also serves as a perfect go-to recipe anytime you're craving a tropical dessert.

+ TARGET DOSE:

About 2.6 mg THC per serving (using Cannabis-Infused Powdered Sugar, page 51)

+ EQUIPMENT:

Blender
Saucepan
Large mixing bowls
Mixer

+ INGREDIENTS:

½ cup dry tapioca pearls

3 cups water

¼ cup mango juice

2 ripe mangoes

⅛ teaspoon finely grounded cardamom

¼ teaspoon puréed ginger

⅛ teaspoon cinnamon

¼ cup sugar

One 6.8-ounce box coconut cream

2 tablespoons Cannabis-Infused Powdered Sugar (page 51)

¼ cup leftover shortbread cookies (page 80) or any vanilla cookie, crumbled

¼ cup toasted pecans

2 tablespoons black sesame seeds

1. In a medium saucepan, cover the dried tapioca pearls with the water; heat on medium-low heat, stirring often. Cook until the tapioca pearls are translucent and you don't see any white dots.
2. Drain the pearls in a strainer, and rinse with cold water until most of the outer starch is rinsed off. Transfer to a bowl.
3. Combine the pearls with the mango juice, and stir thoroughly. Set aside.
4. Purée the mangos in a blender.
5. Add the mango purée, cardamom, ginger, cinnamon, and sugar to a small saucepan; heat on low, occasionally stirring for about 20 minutes or until the mixture has thickened and all ingredients are well incorporated. Turn off heat, and set aside.
6. In a large chilled mixing bowl, whip the coconut cream and powdered sugar until stiff peaks form. (For faster results, pre-chill your coconut cream and repeat until desired consistency is achieved.)
7. Crush the cookies, and add them to a food processor with the toasted pecans. Pulse a few times until the mixture becomes a crumble. Don't overwork it: The pecans will start to become oily like nut butter. Remove to a bowl.
8. Mix the toasted black sesame into the crumble.
9. In a dessert cup, assemble the pudding in layers: first the crumble, then the tapioca pearls, the mango purée, and the coconut whip. Repeat.
10. Add a final sprinkle of crumble on top for presentation.

Tip! We've tried many brands of coconut cream for whipping and found that the Kara brand works best for this recipe. The coconut cream will be extra smooth and creamy, and it will also hold up in the fridge for a day or two in advance without defluffing.

YIELD: 8 SCOOPS (4 OUNCES)

SWEET CORN ICE CREAM

Who doesn't love corn? We know sweet corn might not be a flavor of ice cream you're used to, but trust us: This deliciously unique dessert is sure to spark conversation among your friends. Both sweet and creamy, this ice cream is an interesting blend of flavors that will have you coming back for more! If you're an ice cream lover, it's definitely a new one to try. If you're lucky enough to find fresh sweet corn, nothing beats corn in peak season, but you can always buy a can of sweet corn, especially if you're not confident in cutting corn off the cob. This easy-to-follow recipe can be made without an ice cream maker, but if you have one, skip steps 6 and 7.

+ TARGET DOSE:

About 7.8 mg THC per serving (using Cannabis-Infused Sugar, page 51)

+ EQUIPMENT:

Handheld mixer
Mixing bowls
Measuring cups
Measuring spoons

+ INGREDIENTS:

3 cobs sweet corn, with kernels cut off the cob (about 15 ounces)

2 cups heavy cream

1 cup whole milk

¼ caster sugar

¼ cup Cannabis-Infused Sugar (page 51)

½ tablespoon vanilla extract

Pinch of salt

1. Cut the corn off the cob.
2. Purée the corn in a blender until completely smooth.
3. In a medium saucepan, heat the heavy cream, whole milk, sugars, vanilla extract,, and pinch of salt on medium heat, just until the sugar is dissolved. Be careful not to bring it to a boil.
4. Add the corn purée to the cream, and mix well.
5. Pass the mixture through a strainer to catch any chunks leftover from the corn purée. This is an important step to make sure your ice cream comes out as smooth as possible.
6. Let the mixture cool to room temperature; then cover it and put it in the freezer for 2 hours or until it is semi-frozen.
7. Take the bowl out of the fridge, and use a hand mixer to make it smooth again by breaking up any icicles or other chunks. Alternatively, you can use an ice cream maker, if you have one. Put the ice cream back in the freezer. Repeat this step one more time in an hour.
8. Freeze again for another hour and then enjoy, or transfer the mixture to a freezer-safe container to enjoy later.

YIELD: 4 SERVINGS (4 OUNCES)

TOFU CHOCOLATE PUDDING

When you're in the mood for chocolate pudding, this recipe will be your go-to! (And let's be honest, who isn't ever in the mood for chocolate pudding?) This tofu chocolate pudding is decadent, with a mousse-like texture blended into a dark chocolate dessert. This sweet treat packs a rich cocoa punch to smash any sweet tooth cravings from even the biggest chocolate lovers, but with less guilt. Incredibly easy to make, this simple recipe requires only a few ingredients and limited equipment.

+ TARGET DOSE:

10 mg THC per serving (using Cannabis-Infused Simple Syrup, page 60)

+ EQUIPMENT:

Blender or food processor

Silicone spatula

+ INGREDIENTS:

16-ounce block silken tofu

¼ cup high-quality unsweetened dark chocolate powder

1 tablespoon maple syrup

Pinch of salt

¼ cup Cannabis-Infused Simple Syrup (page 60)

¼ cup caster sugar

1. Wrap the tofu in a paper towel, and place it under something that can apply soft pressure to drain some of the moisture. You can use anything here to apply pressure, such as a hardback book or a jar of soup.
2. Put the drained tofu in a blender, and blend until completely smooth.
3. Add the rest of the ingredients to the tofu mixture. Blend until everything is completely combined. Feel free to adjust the intensity of the chocolate or the sweetness, to your preference.
4. Divide the chocolate pudding into the small dessert bowls to enjoy immediately, or chill in the fridge for later.
5. Optional toppings include whipped cream, fresh berries, toasted almonds, toasted coconut, and butter waffle cookies.

> *Tip!* Get as creative with the toppings as your heart desires. You can also put out a topping bar with multiple options for your guests to customize their own puddings.

YIELD: 12 TO 15 DOUGHNUTS

OOEY GOOEY BANANA DOUGHNUTS WITH PANDAN CONDENSED MILK

The name says it all! These fried banana doughnuts are deliciously ooey and gooey. How often do you have an overly ripe banana sitting in your fruit bowl, begging to be put out of its misery? Give these brown, spotted bananas the decedent makeover they are meant for and dip them in the pandan condensed milk with this next-level fried banana doughnut recipe.

+ TARGET DOSE:

Your preferred dose (using Cannabis-Infused Powdered Sugar, page 51)

+ EQUIPMENT:

Mixing bowls

Heavy bottom pot or wok, for frying

Slotted spoon or spider

Small cookie or ice cream scoop

Wire rack

Duster

+ INGREDIENTS:

2 ripe bananas

1 egg

¼ sugar

¼ cup buttermilk

3 tablespoons unsalted butter, melted

1 teaspoon vanilla extract

1¼ cups all-purpose flour, sifted

2 teaspoons baking powder

½ teaspoon salt

4 cups vegetable oil

Cannabis-Infused Powdered Sugar at your preferred dose (page 51), for dusting

4 to 6 drops pandan syrup

1 cup condensed milk

1. In a small mixing bowl, smash the bananas with a fork until most clumps are gone.
2. Combine the bananas, egg, sugar, buttermilk, melted butter, and vanilla extract until well mixed.
3. In a separate bowl, mix together all the dry ingredients: sifted flour, baking powder, and salt.
4. Gradually fold in the dry ingredients using a silicone spatula until just combined. For the fluffiest results, be sure to not overwork the dough.
5. Heat the vegetable oil in a heavy-bottomed pot (there should be about 2 inches of oil in your pan). Use a baking thermometer to heat the oil until it reaches 325°F (163°C).
6. Use a small cookie scoop or ice cream scoop to form even balls of dough. Drop a few balls into the oil at a time, without overcrowding the pot.
7. Fry the doughnuts until they're golden brown on all sides, about 2 to 3 minutes.
8. Using a spider or a slotted spoon, remove the doughnuts onto some paper towels to drain the excess oil; transfer to a wire rack. Repeat with the remaining batter.
9. Dust with Cannabis-Infused Powdered Sugar, and eat while hot.
10. In a small bowl, combine pandan syrup and condensed milk thoroughly and use as a dipping sauce.

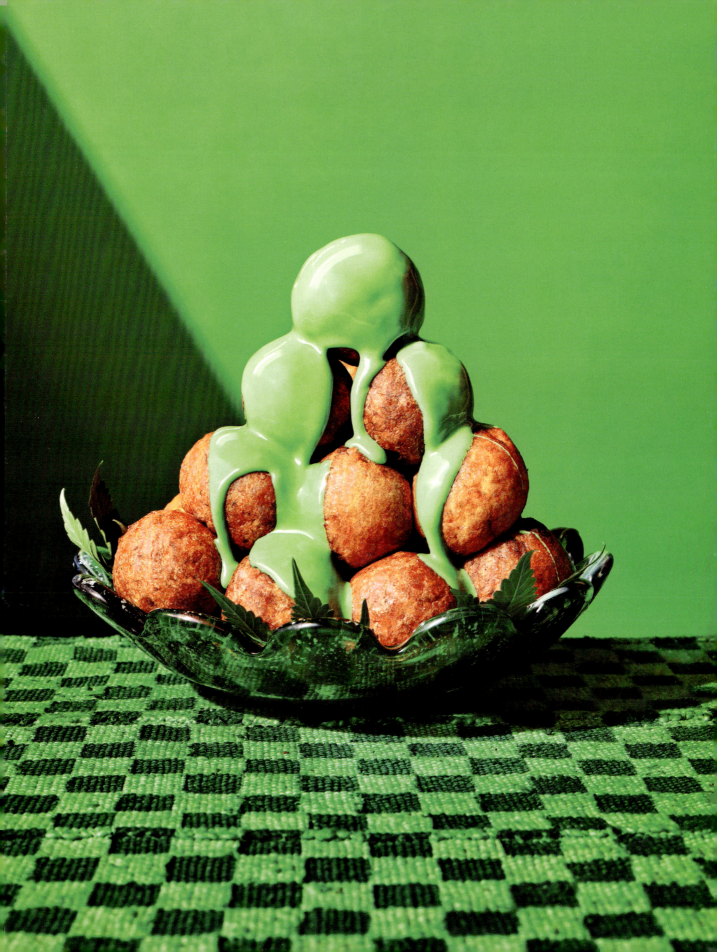

SAVORY EATS

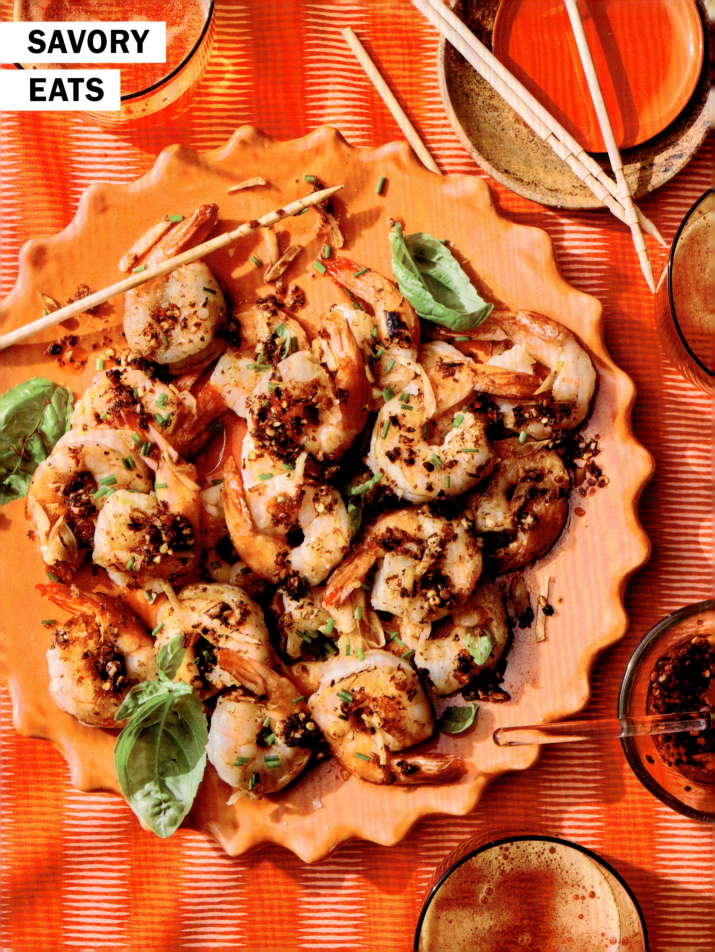

YIELD: 3 SERVINGS (7 TO 8 SHRIMP)

CHILI GARLIC SHRIMP

For the amount of flavor, this is one of the easiest dishes you can make in the least amount of time. Shrimp, butter, and garlic are already an infamous trifecta, but add some Cannabis-Infused Chili Oil, and this recipe will have a depth of flavor that tastes like hours went into preparing it! In truth, this recipe takes only 15 minutes. Make this your go-to when you're in need of a fast and utterly flavorful meal.

+ TARGET DOSE:

8 mg THC per serving (using Cannabis-Infused Chili Oil, page 47)

+ EQUIPMENT:

Large skillet

+ INGREDIENTS:

2 tablespoons avocado oil

1 pound large shrimp (21 to 25 per pound in size), peeled and deveined

¼ cup butter

4 tablespoons garlic, chopped

Pinch of black pepper

¼ teaspoon salt

1 teaspoon lemon juice

2 tablespoons Cannabis-Infused Chili Oil (page 47)

3 tablespoons chives (or whichever fresh herb you like, such as basil, parsley, or cilantro)

1. On medium-high heat, in a large skillet, add the avocado oil and the shrimp. Cook for about 1 minute on each side.
2. Lower the heat to medium. Add the butter, garlic, and pepper to the pan, and toss with the shrimp. Let cook for about 2 minutes.
3. Add the salt, lemon juice, and Cannabis-Infused Chili Oil to the shrimp, and toss. Top with chives, and enjoy immediately.

YIELD: ABOUT 15 TO 20 WINGS

BIG BAD FRIED CHICKEN

Korean fried chicken, also known as KFC, has become a global icon. Different from American fried chicken, this fried chicken is twice-fried in a starch-based dry batter, which creates an ultra-crisp and light texture. The glazes you can use to sauce your fried chicken are endless, but soy or gochujang (chili paste) sauces are the most popular.

+ TARGET DOSE:

About 1.6 to 1.2 mg THC per wing (using Cannabis-Infused Coconut Oil, page 44)

+ EQUIPMENT:

Thermometer

Parchment paper

Heavy-bottomed or cast-iron pot

Mixing bowls

Measuring spoons

Measuring cups

Wire rack

Silicone spatula

+ INGREDIENTS:

1½ pounds chicken wings

1 cup cornstarch

½ teaspoon baking powder

1 tablespoon onion powder

¼ teaspoon salt

¼ teaspoon pepper

1 tablespoon Cannabis-Infused Coconut Oil (page 44)

2 tablespoons chopped jalapeños

2 tablespoons ginger

2 tablespoons garlic

2 tablespoons scallions, chopped

1 teaspoon soy sauce

3 tablespoons fish sauce

¼ cup honey

2 tablespoons brown sugar

¼ teaspoon black pepper

1. Thoroughly pat dry the chicken wings with a paper towel, removing as much excess moisture as possible.
2. Space out the wings on a sheet tray lined with parchment paper. Put the wings in the fridge, uncovered, to dry out for at least 3 hours (or overnight).
3. Before you start frying, remove the chicken from the fridge and let it sit at room temperature for about 30 minutes.
4. Combine the cornstarch, baking powder, onion powder, salt, and pepper in a bowl. Set aside.
5. In a medium saucepan on low heat, add the Cannabis-Infused Coconut Oil, and sauté the jalapeños, ginger, garlic, and scallions until tender. Add in the soy sauce, fish sauce, brown sugar, honey, and pepper until the mixture is thickened and bubbling, stirring occasionally. Remove from heat.
6. In a heavy-bottomed or cast-iron pot, add enough oil for frying, about 2 inches. Using a thermometer, bring the temperature to about 350°F (176°C).
7. Thoroughly coat each chicken wing with the cornstarch mixture, pressing the dry batter onto the wing.
8. Carefully and gently drop the wings into the oil, making sure not to overcrowd the pot. Keep the temperature at a consistent 325°F (163°C) for about 5 to 7 minutes.
9. Transfer the wings to a rack, and repeat with the rest of the chicken in however many batches are necessary. Once you've fried all your wings, they're ready for their second fry.
10. This time, bring your oil to 375°F (190°C), and double-fry the wings for about 1 to 2 minutes more.
11. Transfer the wings to a wire rack and let the excess oil drain off.
12. In a giant mixing bowl, toss the fried chicken with the fish sauce glaze you made, add a pinch of salt, and enjoy while hot and crispy!

> **Tip!** Frying your wings twice is crucial to getting that signature Korean Fried Chicken crisp on these wings, so don't skip this step!

YIELD: 4 SERVINGS

BRAISED SHORT RIBS

Always a staple during holidays or family gatherings, this recipe for galbi-jjim, or Korean braised short ribs, is a hearty main dish. Although it takes a few hours for the meat to get tender, once you have it in the pot, you can set the heat to simmer and let the meat do its thing. The longer you braise, the more tender it will be. We recommend going low and slow so it retains all the moisture of the beef while rendering out the fat. Fall-off-the-bone amazing, here we come!

+ TARGET DOSE:
10 mg THC per serving (using Cannabis-Infused Sugar, page 51)

+ EQUIPMENT:
Large pot
Measuring cups
Measuring spoons

+ INGREDIENTS:
4 pounds short ribs (bone in), cut into 3-inch pieces
2 cups soy sauce
1½ cups brown sugar
2 tablespoons black pepper
3 tablespoons minced ginger
2 tablespoons chopped garlic
2 tablespoons mirin
3 star anise
1 cup orange juice
1 cup water
2 teaspoons Cannabis-Infused Sugar (page 51)
½ cup rice wine
2 chopped onions
3 chopped carrots
2 medium chopped potatoes
Toasted sesame seeds, for garnish
Scallions, for garnish

1. Soak your short ribs in cold water for at least an hour to draw out the blood from the meat. Set aside.
2. In a large pot, combine the soy sauce, brown sugar, black pepper, ginger, garlic, mirin, star anise, orange juice, water, infused sugar, and rice wine. Bring to a boil.
3. Pat the short ribs dry with a paper towel. Sear all sides on high heat for 1 minute in a large skillet. Add the seared meat to the sauce.
4. Set the heat to a low simmer, and add your short ribs. Cover with a lid, and cook for at least 3 hours. Use a fork to check for your desired tenderness.
5. When you're about 30 minutes to an hour away from your meat being done, add in the vegetables, and cook for 3 to 5 hours, to your desired tenderness.
6. Garnish with some toasted sesame seeds and scallions, and serve family style.

Tip! **If you like the sauce a little thicker, mix 2 teaspoons cornstarch with 1 tablespoon cold water in a small bowl until no clumps remain, and add to your pot of short ribs. Stir in immediately.**

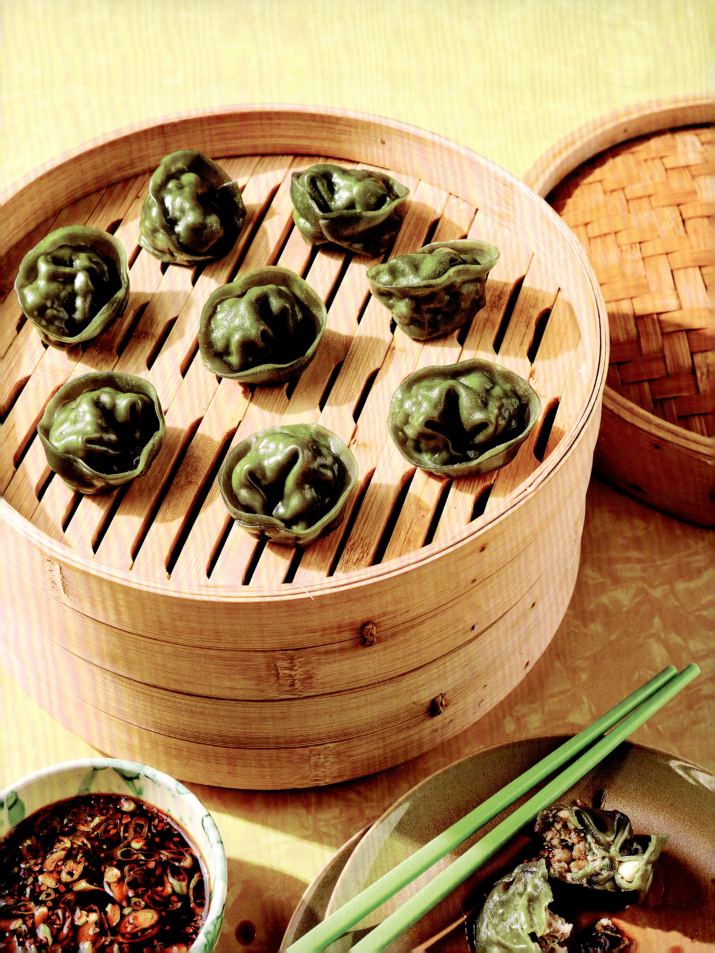

YIELD: 15 TO 20 DUMPLINGS

JUICED CANNA LEAF DUMPLINGS

Who doesn't love a plump and juicy dumpling? We certainly do! These Korean-style dumplings, or *mandu*, are perfect mouthwatering pockets of meat-filled joy. We swapped out a traditional flour-and-water dumpling wrapper for this version, using juiced cannabis fan leaves. Like most leafy greens, they have a ton of nutritional benefits, but they also add a subtle herbaceous flavor to your dumplings. Be sure to serve with the dipping sauce, and don't be shy—you'll want to devour these!

+ TARGET DOSE:
About 0.5 mg THC per teaspoon of dipping sauce (using Cannabis-Infused Simple Syrup, page 60)

+ EQUIPMENT:
Rolling pin
Large mixing bowl
Juicer
Digital scale

+ INGREDIENTS:

For the dumpling wrappers:
1 cup all-purpose flour
¼ teaspoon salt
2 tablespoons warm water
¼ cup juiced cannabis fan leaves (found online, or substitute spinach juice)

For the filling:
½ pound ground pork
½ pound chopped, peeled, and deveined shrimp
1 teaspoon grated ginger
½ teaspoon garlic
¼ cup diced shiitake mushrooms
¼ cup chopped chives or scallions
1 tablespoon soy sauce
½ tablespoon fish sauce
1 teaspoon white pepper
Pinch of salt
1 egg
½ tablespoon flour
¼ teaspoon sesame oil

For the dipping sauce:
3 tablespoons soy sauce
2 tablespoons black or rice vinegar
½ tablespoon Korean chili flakes
½ tablespoon sesame
½ tablespoon scallions
3 teaspoons Cannabis-Infused Simple Syrup (page 60)

Recipe continued on page 120

1. To make the dumpling wrappers, mix together the flour, salt, water, and cannabis juice on a clean work surface. Knead the cannabis leaf dough for about 3 minutes until it becomes smooth and elastic. Cover with a clean, damp towel, and set aside for at least 20 to 30 minutes.

2. In the meantime, get started on the filling. In a large mixing bowl, combine the pork, shrimp, ginger, garlic, shiitake mushrooms, chives or scallions, soy sauce, fish sauce, white pepper, a pinch of salt, flour, and the sesame oil. While wearing food-safe gloves, thoroughly mix everything together, or use a stand mixer. You want to ensure that everything is well incorporated.

3. Divide the dough into small golf ball–size balls (about 30 grams or 1 ounce), using a scale to ensure evenly sized dumplings.

4. Using a rolling pin, roll out each dough ball into a circle. This part takes a while to master, but nothing beats fresh dumpling wrappers; stick with it, if you can. (Of course, you can always use store-bought wrappers and skip steps 1 and 3.)

5. Prepare a small bowl of fresh water. Place a small spoonful of filling in the middle of each wrapper. (Beginners tend to overfill their dumplings, making it harder to seal. Figuring out the right amount is key, but it could take a few tries.) Dip your finger in the water bowl, and trace the moisture along the edges of the wrapper. Then fold the wrapper in half, and pinch the edges together. There are so many fancy variations of pleating, crimping, and sealing your dumplings, but a simple half-moon shape is an easy place to start your dumpling journey.

6. You have two options for cooking your dumplings:

Boiled dumplings:

1. Bring a large pot of water to a boil. Drop in the dumplings, and cook for about 5 to 7 minutes or until all the dumplings easily float to the top and the filling is cooked through.

Pan-fried dumplings:

1. Heat 2 tablespoons of oil in a nonstick pan with a lid. Add the dumplings to the pan, and cook on high heat for about 1 minute. Pour ¼ cup of water into the pan, and cover with the lid (so the dumplings can steam while also pan frying); cook on medium heat until all the water has disappeared. Add 1 more tablespoon of oil, and cook on high heat again for another few minutes.

2. For the dipping sauce, combine all the sauce ingredients in a small bowl; mix together until well combined.

3. Serve the dumplings while hot and juicy, with the dipping sauce on the side.

> *Tip!* If you have a hard time finding fresh cannabis leaves, you can use spinach juice instead of cannabis juice to get the same beautiful green color. If you make more dumplings than you can eat in one sitting, don't worry: These hold well in the freezer, so you can take them out and enjoy them whenever you want. Either cooking method works for these frozen dumplings; they'll just take a little more time to cook all the way through.

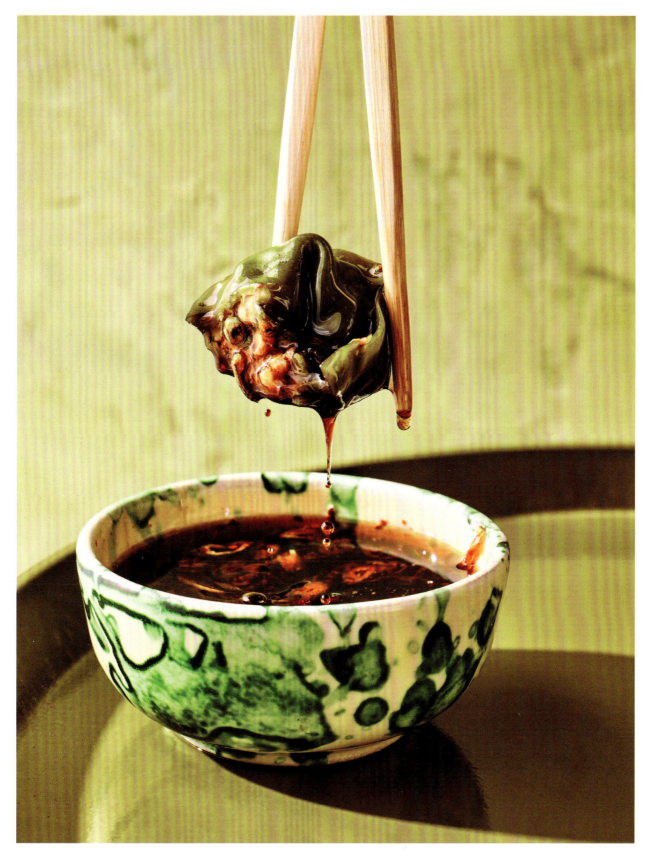

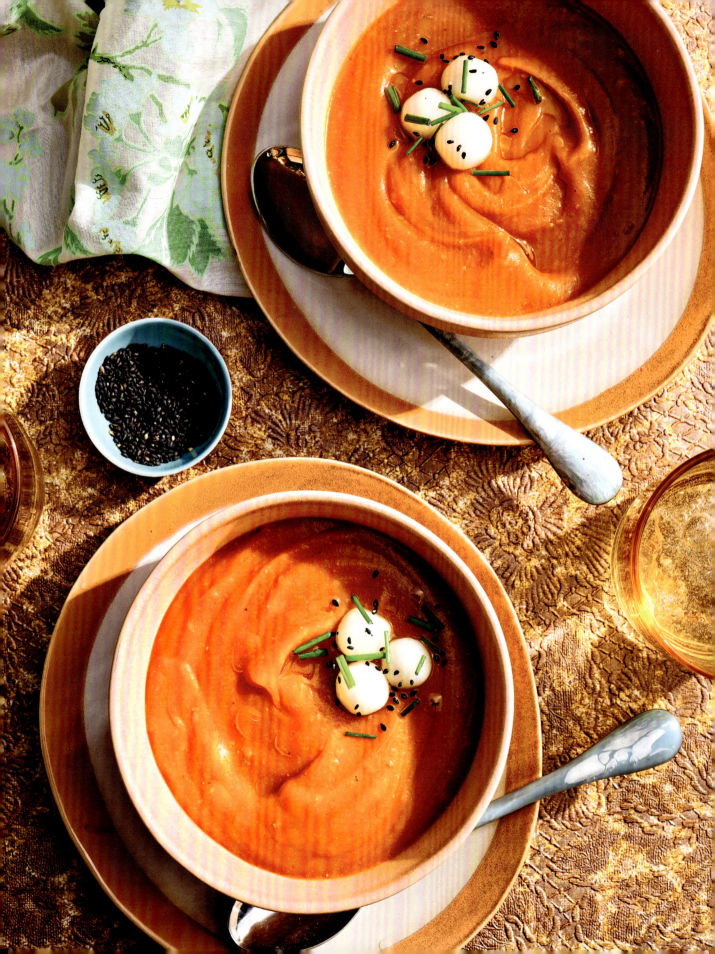

YIELD: 3 BOWLS

KABOCHA PUMPKIN JOOK WITH MOCHI

When it's cold and rainy outside, there's nothing better than kabocha pumpkin jook with mochi. This soup is the ultimate comfort food that wraps you in the biggest, warmest hug. If you've never tasted this soup, you're going to love the texture: It's made with tiny balls of chewy rice flour mochi. Whether you're feeling under the weather or you simply want something to warm the body and soul, this recipe is the best way to cozy up on any cold day.

+ TARGET DOSE:

Your preferred dose (using Cannabis-Infused Olive Oil, page 44)

+ EQUIPMENT:

Blender or handheld immersion blender

Pot

Steamer

+ INGREDIENTS:

For the soup:

2 pounds kabocha pumpkin

3 cups dashi or vegetable stock

2 tablespoons tomato paste

Pinch of black pepper

Pinch of anise powder

¼ teaspoon fish sauce (optional)

1 tablespoon puréed ginger

Pinch of cardamom

1 tablespoon honey

1 cup sweet rice flour

¼ water

1 teaspoon sesame oil

Pinch of salt

½ teaspoon salt

For the garnish:

Drizzle of Cannabis-Infused Olive Oil at your preferred dose (page 44)

Crackle of fresh black pepper

1. Peel and section the kabocha pumpkin into quarters, and place it in a pot with a steamer basket. Steam on medium-high heat for about 25 minutes until the pumpkin is fork tender.

2. When cool enough to touch, transfer the pumpkin and dashi to a blender and purée until smooth (or use an immersion blender, and purée in the pot).

3. Bring the purée back up to medium heat. Add the tomato paste, black pepper, anise powder, fish sauce (if desired), ginger, cardamom, and honey. Simmer on low for another 20 minutes so that all the aromatics and spices infuse into the soup.

4. Combine the rice flour and water in a bowl, and work into a pastelike consistency. Roll into small balls.

5. Bring a small pot filled half way with water to a boil. Drop the rice balls into the water, and swirl them around. They should be done in about 1 to 2 minutes.

6. Rinse the excess starch off the mochi in a cool water bath (no ice). Using a slotted spoon, transfer the mochi into a bowl, removing as much water as possible. Drizzle with a teaspoon of sesame oil and a pinch of salt.

7. Ladle your soup into a bowl, add 4 to 6 mochi, drizzle them with Cannabis-Infused Olive Oil, and a crackle fresh black pepper, and serve.

> *Tip!* When choosing a kabocha pumpkin, you want to look for something heavy for its size. It should be dark green with a bright orange mark.

YIELD: 8 TO 10 PANCAKES

KOREAN VEGGIE PANCAKES

Growing up, these pancakes were a weekly staple in my household. There are so many variations on this snack, with a crispy exterior and a soft and chewy interior. You might be familiar with the seafood or kimchi pancake, but these snacks are so versatile. My family and I ended up adding whatever veggies we needed to use up in the fridge! I've had so many different Korean pancakes in my life, but there's nothing like the ones you grew up with. The following is a recipe for my mom's classic veggie pancakes.

+ TARGET DOSE:

About 0.5 mg THC per teaspoon of dipping sauce (using Cannabis-Infused Simple Syrup, page 60)

+ EQUIPMENT:

Large mixing bowl

Nonstick pan

+ INGREDIENTS:

For the pancakes:

1 cup all-purpose flour

1 cup cold water

1 teaspoon salt

½ teaspoon white pepper

¼ cup julienne onion

½ cup julienne zucchini

½ cup chopped chives or scallions

¼ cup julienne sweet potato

½ cup julienne carrots

Vegetable oil, for cooking

For the dipping sauce:

3 tablespoons soy sauce

2 tablespoons black or rice vinegar

½ tablespoon Korean chili flakes

½ tablespoon sesame

½ tablespoon scallions

3 teaspoons Cannabis-Infused Simple Syrup (page 60)

1. In a large mixing bowl, add the flour, water, salt, and pepper. Mix until smooth.
2. Add all the vegetables in the ingredients list to the flour mixture, and stir until thoroughly combined.
3. Heat 2 tablespoons vegetable oil in a nonstick pan over medium heat.
4. Use a ladle to add the veggie pancake batter to the hot pan, and spread out as evenly as possible.
5. Cook for about 3 minutes or until crispy and golden brown.
6. Flip the pancakes, and cook for another 2 to 3 minutes or until crispy and golden brown. Repeat with the remaining batter.
7. For the dipping sauce, combine all the sauce ingredients in a small bowl, and mix together until well combined.
8. Serve hot off the pan, with the dipping sauce on the side.

YIELD: 8 SERVINGS (20 GRAPE HALVES)

QUICK KIMCHI COTTON CANDY GRAPES

Did you know there are hundreds of different types of kimchi? Well, we're adding kimchi grapes to that list! If you're lucky enough to come across cotton candy grapes, we highly recommend them in this recipe. They're seedless, they have a great crisp to their bite, and they're super sweet and juicy. These grapes are the perfect accompaniment to so many dishes, but you'll often catch us eating them by themselves, standing with the fridge open. They're that good!

+ TARGET DOSE:

7.5 mg THC per serving (using Cannabis-Infused Sugar, page 51)

+ EQUIPMENT:

Mixing bowl

Measuring spoons

+ INGREDIENTS:

1 tablespoon minced garlic

½ tablespoon minced ginger

½ tablespoon fish sauce

2 tablespoons chives

2 tablespoons rice wine vinegar

1 tablespoon Cannabis-Infused Sugar (page 51)

1 pound cotton candy grapes (about 80 grapes)

⅛ teaspoon sea salt

3 tablespoons Korean chile flakes

½ teaspoon sesame oil

1. To make the kimchi mixture, combine the minced garlic, ginger, fish sauce, chives, vinegar, and infused sugar in a small bowl. It should be a pastelike consistency.
2. Cut the grapes in half and combine them with the kimchi mixture.
3. Add a pinch of sea salt. Toss and enjoy!

Tip! This kimchi mixture can work on so many different vegetables and fruits: tomatoes, cucumbers, and more. If you're a kimchi lover, have fun experimenting with what you find at your local produce shop

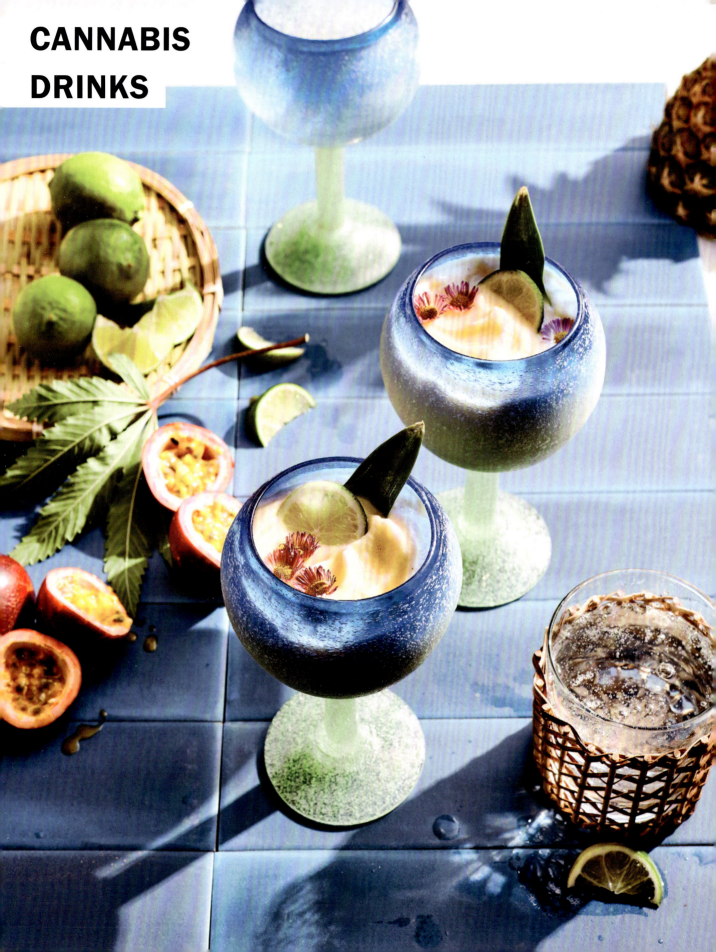

CANNABIS DRINKS

YIELD: 1 SERVING

PASSION FRUIT CANNA-COLADA

When it comes to piña coladas, there isn't a more perfect drink to pair with endless days of sunshine. To keep your palate refreshed during the warmer months, our spin on this classic cocktail contains passion fruit juice, cannabis-infused coconut milk, cream of coconut, lime juice, and a splash of fat-washed coconut rum (if you're feeling a little naughty). Both tangy and sweet, this creamy blended drink is hard to resist and will instantly transport your taste buds to a tropical destination, no matter where you reside. Since you're using frozen pineapple, you can skip adding ice to this recipe. By using frozen fruit, you'll prevent the drink from getting watered down.

+ TARGET DOSE:

8 mg to 10 mg THC | < 1 mg CBD per drink (using Cannabis-Infused Coconut Milk, page 62, and optional Fat-Washed Coconut Rum, page 68) or your preferred dose (using a commercially made THC tincture of your choice, see note below)

+ EQUIPMENT:

Blender

12-ounce drinking glass of your choice

Spice grater

+ INGREDIENTS:

2 cups frozen pineapple

3 ounces (90 mL) passion fruit juice

½ ounce (15 mL) Cannabis-Infused Coconut Milk (page 62)

½ ounce (15 mL) coconut milk

3 tablespoons cream of coconut

½ ounce (15 mL) freshly squeezed lime juice

¾ ounce (22 mL) Fat-Washed Coconut Rum (optional, see page 68)

1 whole nutmeg

Pineapple leaf, a pineapple slice, a lime wedge, and a pink edible flower for garnish

1. Combine the frozen pineapple, passion fruit juice, Cannabis-Infused Coconut Milk, coconut milk, cream of coconut, lime juice, and Fat-Washed Coconut Rum (if using) in the bottom of a blender.
2. Blend on high until the drink is smooth and creamy.
3. Pour the canna-colada into a drinking glass of your choice; then use a spice grater to grate a sprinkle of fresh nutmeg on top of the drink.
4. Garnish, and if you have fresh-cut cannabis leaves on hand, add a leaf for some extra flair; serve immediately.

> *Tip!* If you don't have time to create Cannabis-Infused Coconut Milk, you can easily infuse this recipe by using the THC or CBD tincture of your choice (even if it's oil based). Simply swap the infused coconut milk for regular coconut milk, add the tincture to the bottom of the blender in step 1 with the other ingredients, and blend away. When preparing this recipe, the best cream of coconut to use is produced by Coco Lopez, a classic addition for the best piña coladas! See "Resources" on page 169 for other ingredient recommendations.

YIELD: 1 SERVING

GINGER PEACH CREAMSICLE SMOOTHIE

One of the best ways to start the day is to blend up a delicious cannabis-infused smoothie. If you're a fan of ginger, this Ginger Peach Creamsicle Smoothie might be your new go-to. By adding fresh ginger mixed with cannabis, this smoothie helps battle inflammation to jumpstart your system while also enchanting the palate with creamy peach notes. Infused with canna-honey and supercharged with vanilla protein powder, this smoothie is seriously delicious and filling. For best results, use frozen fruit to create a thick texture—you'll want to eat this with a spoon!

+ TARGET DOSE:

4 mg to 8 mg THC | 0 mg CBD per drink (using Cannabis-Infused Honey, page 50) or your preferred dose (using commercially made cannabis-infused honey of your choice)

+ EQUIPMENT:

Blender

Glass of your choice

+ INGREDIENTS:

¾ cup frozen peaches

¾ cup frozen banana slices

1 heaping teaspoon fresh ginger, cut into pieces (add more if you like it extra gingery)

4 ounces (120 mL) orange juice

2 ounces (60 mL) milk of your choice (for this recipe, we used oat milk)

1 to 2 teaspoons Cannabis-Infused Honey (page 50)

1 scoop vanilla protein powder

Peach slice, for garnish

1. Add all the ingredients to a blender.
2. Blend until smooth and creamy, and then fill a serving glass of your choice.
3. Garnish with a slice of peach.

> *Tip!* If you haven't prepared the Cannabis-Infused Honey and you don't have a commercially made cannabis honey at home, you can still incorporate THC or CBD into this recipe by adding your favorite unflavored tincture (at your preferred dose) into the blender. Simply blend with the other ingredients, and enjoy.

YIELD: 1 SERVING

PEANUT BUTTER HOT CHOCOLATE

When it's cold outside and you're craving something decadent, look no further than a cannabis-infused Peanut Butter Hot Chocolate! This creamy, chocolatey, and deliciously warm beverage will satisfy your sweet tooth, as well as provide a boost of phytocannabinoids and other healing cannabis compounds. Made with peanut butter chips, semisweet chocolate chips, a dash of Cannabis-Infused Coconut Milk, plus other flavorful ingredients, this drink is a mouthwatering treat to enjoy—plus, it's so easy to make. Spoil yourself by topping the drink with a sprinkle of chopped mini peanut butter cups—you deserve it!

+ TARGET DOSE:

5 mg to 10 mg THC | < 1 mg CBD per drink (using Cannabis-Infused Coconut Milk, page 62) or your preferred dose (using a commercially made cannabis-infused chocolate bar of your choice—see the note below)

+ EQUIPMENT:

Measuring cups

Small saucepan

Rubber spatula

Whisk

Mug of your choice

+ INGREDIENTS:

⅛ cup (16 grams) semisweet chocolate chips

¼ cup (32 grams) peanut butter chips

8 ounces (236 mL) milk (I prefer 2 percent dairy milk with this recipe, but use what you'd like)

¼ teaspoon vanilla extract

Pinch of sea salt

½ ounce (15 mL) or your preferred dose Cannabis-Infused Coconut Milk (page 62)

Garnish with a dollop of whipped cream and chopped mini peanut butter cups

1. Begin by heating the chocolate chips and peanut butter chips in the bottom of a small saucepan. Keep the temperature on low heat, to prevent burning.
2. Continuously stir with a rubber spatula until the chocolate and peanut butter pieces melt completely and no lumps remain. Continue to heat until well combined.
3. Turn the heat to medium, and slowly stir in the milk, the vanilla extract, and a pinch of sea salt. Continue to stir the blend until it reaches 180°F (82°C) (or slightly simmering, but do not boil).
4. Scrape the sides of the saucepan with a rubber spatula; then use a whisk to combine the melted chocolate and peanut butter with the other ingredients. Whisk until the blend is smooth and consistent—the heated milk should look smooth and creamy.
5. Remove from heat, and then whisk in the Cannabis-Infused Coconut Milk to infuse the drink.
6. Pour into a mug of your choice, and top with whipped cream and a sprinkle of chopped mini peanut butter cups. Serve warm, and enjoy!

Tip! If you don't have time to prepare the Cannabis-Infused Coconut Milk, you can easily infuse this recipe by substituting the semisweet chocolate chips for one serving (or your preferred dose) of your favorite commercially made cannabis-infused chocolate bar available at your local licensed dispensary. Melt the cannabis chocolate with the peanut butter chips in step 1, and then follow the recipe as directed. Using a commercially made chocolate ensures that this drink will be precisely dosed.

YIELD: 1 SERVING

BLOOD ORANGE RASPBERRY SOUR

When blood oranges are in season, this is the perfect spirit-free recipe to celebrate with! Made with freshly squeezed blood orange juice muddled with lime juice and fresh raspberries, this mouthwatering drink glows with a bright red hue (but be careful—it stains!). Infused with both cannabis fruit syrup *and* a dash of cannabis bitters, this highly elevated drink is a stunner, complete with a raspberry-dusted cannabis leaf on top of the froth. To create the best foam, be sure to dry shake, and then shake again as directed. This show-stopping recipe is ideal for parties when you'd like to impress friends or family with your creative mixology skills.

+ TARGET DOSE:

10 to 13 mg THC | < 1 mg CBD per drink (using Cannabis-Infused Fruit Syrup, page 64, and Cannabis-Infused Bitters [if using], page 56) or your preferred dose (using a commercially made THC tincture of your choice)

+ EQUIPMENT:

Chilled sour glass

Shaker tin

Muddler

Hawthorn strainer

Fine-mesh strainer

Powder shaker

Cannabis leaf stencil

+ INGREDIENTS:

3 ounces (90 mL) freshly squeezed (or cold-pressed) blood orange juice, with pulp removed

1¼ ounces (37.5 mL) freshly squeezed lime juice

⅓ cup (55.4 grams) fresh raspberries

¼ to ½ ounce (7.5 mL to 15 mL) Cannabis-Infused Fruit Syrup, page 64; feel free to adjust based on the sweetness of the blood orange juice

Dash of aromatic bitters (flip to the Resources on page 169 for our favorite) or, for an enhancement, 1 dash (6 to 8 drops) Cannabis-Infused Bitters (page 56)

1 egg white

Garnish with pulverized Freeze-Dried Raspberry Powdered Sugar (seeds removed), for garnish see page 131

1. Chill a sour glass by placing it in the freezer.

2. While the glass is chilling, add the blood orange juice, lime juice, and raspberries to the bottom of a shaker tin.

3. Muddle the ingredients together for 1 to 2 minutes, to extract as much juice, color, and flavor as possible.

4. Finely strain out the solids, and pour the liquid back into the cleaned shaker. Discard the solids.

5. Add the Cannabis-Infused Fruit Syrup, the Cannabis-Infused Bitters, and the egg white. Cover and dry shake (no ice) for 15 seconds. Add ice, and shake again for 15 seconds or until very cold.

6. Using a Hawthorn strainer, strain the liquid over the chilled sour glass. Shake the strainer to capture as much froth as possible without filling it to the brim.

Recipe continued on page 131

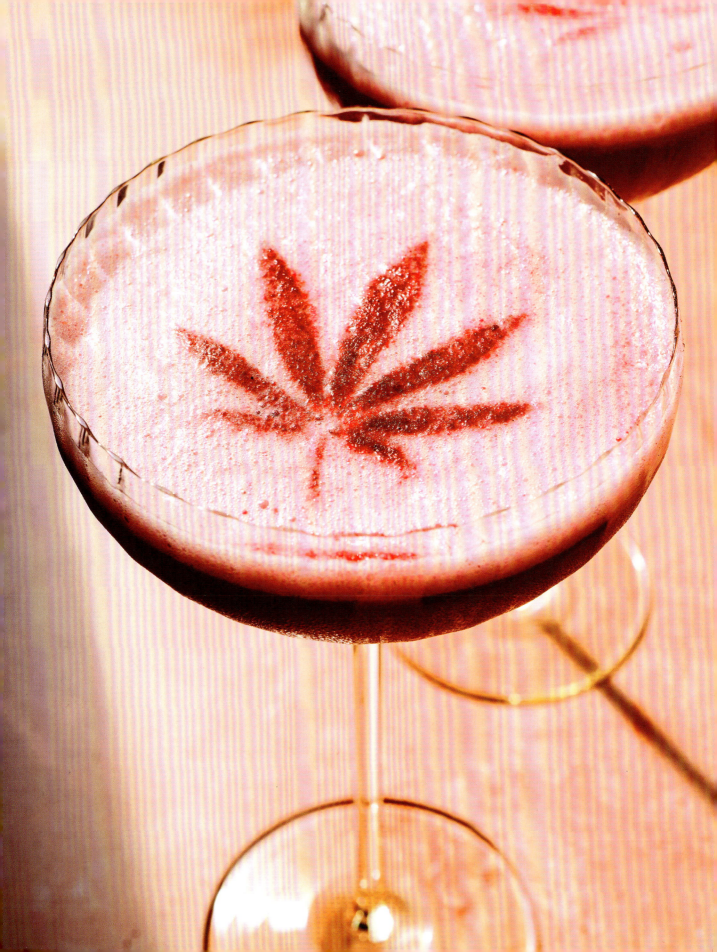

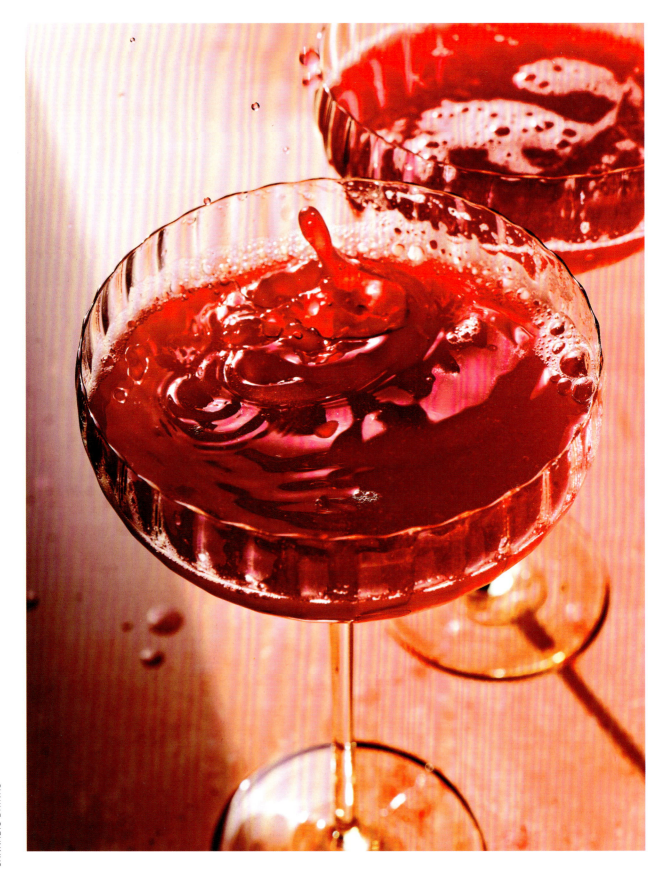

7. Using a cannabis stencil, place the stencil over the top of the glass, and then dust the top of the glass with Pulverized Freeze-Dried Raspberry Powdered Sugar to create a weed leaf garnish.

8. Serve immediately, and enjoy!

How to Make Pulverized Freeze-Dried Raspberry Powdered Sugar

1. Add ⅓ cup freeze-dried raspberries to a spice grinder.
2. Add ½ teaspoon powdered sugar, and blend until it forms a fine powder.
3. Sift into a fine-mesh powder shaker, making sure to remove the raspberry seeds. Cover the shaker, and then shake on top of drinks or desserts.

> **Tip!** If you don't have time to infuse the simple syrup or bitters, simply substitute for the noninfused versions and add your favorite unflavored tincture (at your preferred dose) to the shaker tin before dry shaking. Then proceed with the recipe as noted. An alcohol-based tincture works best.

Tips & Precautions When Mixing Cannabis & Alcohol

As you've learned throughout this book, using alcohol to extract phytocannabinoids is a reliable way to create tinctures and other bar panty items. However, you need to keep some important points in mind as you begin to mix cannabis with cocktails and other alcoholic beverages. Because cannabis and alcohol both produce intoxicating effects that hit stronger when combined, you should always keep safe and responsible consumption in mind. Moderation is key to an enjoyable experience. When preparing cannabis drinks that contain alcohol, always stay below 10 milligrams THC per drink (or between 1 and 2.5 milligrams of THC for beginners), and do not consume more than one unless you are very experienced at consuming both at the same time. Know your limits. Also remember to be patient! Sometimes it can take an hour or more to feel the effects of the cannabis you've consumed. Start low, go slow, and don't overdo it. Otherwise, you might end up feeling dizzy and sick.

When it comes to CBD, it's been noted that alcohol can potentially cancel out the effects of cannabidiol due to the ways these substances interact when consumed together. If you're looking to create solely CBD drinks, I recommend sticking to nonalcoholic drink options.

Last but not least, you should never mix cannabis-infused cocktails with other medications, and definitely never drive or operate machinery after consuming. *Always drink responsibly*!

YIELD: 1 SERVING

BROWN BUTTER OLD FASHIONED

If you're a fan of whiskey, you're going to love this decadent, delicious, and oh-so-buttery Brown Butter Old Fashioned. This out-of-this-world tasty canna-cocktail blends together the cannabis-infused fat-washed brown butter bourbon you created in Chapter 2 (Brown Butter–Washed Bourbon, page 69), along with brown sugar simple syrup and bitters to create a rich and opulent drink that's meant to be savored. Although other sugars can be used in an old fashioned, we love using brown sugar simple syrup with this recipe to add more complex notes and depth to the flavor. If you'd rather skip the alcohol, don't worry: You can still create this recipe with some modifications (see the note on page 134).

+ TARGET DOSE:

5 to 9 mg THC | 0 mg CBD per drink (using Brown Butter–Washed Bourbon, page 69) or your preferred dose (using a commercially made alcohol-based tincture of your choice—see the note on page 134

+ EQUIPMENT:

Measuring cups

Small saucepan

Mixing glass

Bar spoon

Old fashioned glass

Cocktail pick

+ INGREDIENTS:

For the brown sugar simple syrup:

1 cup packed brown sugar

1 cup water

For the old fashioned:

¼ to ½ ounce (7.4 mL to 14.8 mL) brown sugar simple syrup (use ¼ ounce if you prefer a stronger bourbon flavor [it's less sweet, but the brown sugar does add great depth])

1½ ounces (44.3 mL) Brown Butter–Washed Bourbon (page 69)

½ ounce (14.8 mL) bourbon

3 dashes aromatic bitters (flip to page 169 for our favorite)

1 large ice cube

Garnish with a Brown Sugar–Coated Dehydrated Orange Round (page 134) and a Luxardo cherry

Recipe continued on page 136

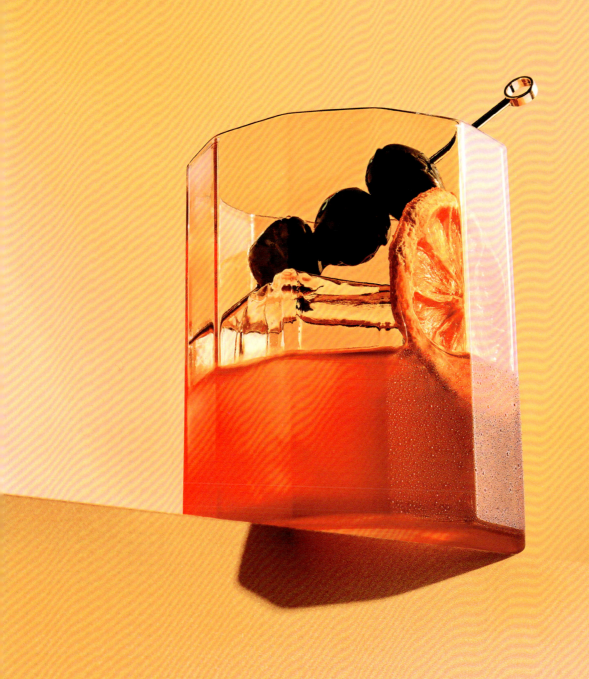

1. Begin by preparing the brown sugar simple syrup. Add 1 cup packed brown sugar and 1 cup water to a small saucepan. Begin to heat over medium heat, constantly stirring until the sugar dissolves into the water. Remove from heat, and then let cool to room temperature.
2. In a mixing glass, combine the Brown Butter–Washed Bourbon, noninfused bourbon, brown sugar simple syrup, and bitters. Stir using a bar spoon, add ice, and then stir again until the bourbon is chilled.
3. Strain into an old fashioned glass containing one large ice cube.
4. Garnish with a Brown Sugar–Coated Dehydrated Orange Round (it's edible!) and a Luxardo cherry on a cocktail pick.

How to Make Brown Sugar–Coated Dehydrated Orange Rounds

1. Preheat the oven to 225°F (107°C). While the oven is heating, cut an orange into round slices, leaving the peel on.
2. Coat both sides of the orange using your desired amount of brown sugar. Place the rounds on a baking rack or cooling rack on top of a baking sheet.
3. Bake for 2 hours; then flip, and bake for another 2 hours.
4. Remove from heat, let cool, and use as a decorative cocktail garnish or dip into melted chocolate to make a tasty dessert treat.

> *Tip!* If you'd rather infuse this recipe using a commercially made tincture, prepare the Brown Butter–Washed Bourbon (page 69) using noninfused butter and then add the tincture to the mixing glass during step 1. Just make sure you're using an alcohol-based tincture so that it blends with the other liquids without separating (in other words, avoid using an oil-based tincture). If you'd rather skip the alcohol altogether and create a mocktail, use a whiskey-flavored nonalcoholic spirit, and infuse the brown sugar simple syrup with cannabis instead of creating a fat-wash infusion. Just be aware that you'll be making more of a traditional old fashioned instead of a Brown Butter Old Fashioned. Refer to page 60 for a Cannabis-Infused Simple Syrup recipe.

YIELD: 1 SERVING

DETOX JUICE

For a boost of THCA or CBDA, one of the best ways to access these nonintoxicating phytocannabinoids is to prepare a fresh canna-leaf juice. Similar to the traditional "green juice," this invigorating farm-to-table recipe is a fantastic way to integrate a wealth of nutrients into your daily routine. To make this a detox juice, add a teaspoon of flaxseed oil, which will get your digestive tract moving (as well as add fiber to your diet).

+ TARGET DOSE:

Nonintoxicating THCA and CBDA

+ EQUIPMENT:

Juicer

Mason jar

+ INGREDIENTS:

2 to 3 handfuls fresh cannabis leaves (or 4 full kale leaves)

1 chilled lemon, cut into quarters and peeled

One 1-inch piece fresh ginger, peeled and sliced in half (add more if you love fresh ginger notes)

½ English cucumber

1 chilled Honeycrisp apple (or whatever variety of apple you prefer), cut into slices

1 teaspoon flaxseed oil

1. Feed the cannabis leaves (or kale), lemon, ginger, cucumber, and apple into a juicer, altering the ingredients as you continue to juice.
2. Once everything is juiced, add the flaxseed oil to the liquid; stir to combine.
3. Pour the juice into a serving glass of your choice, and enjoy immediately. This recipe yields about 16 ounces, so it could serve two, but if you're like us, you'll drink the entire thing!

Tip! **The best way to source fresh cannabis leaves is to grow your own plants. However, if you can't access fresh cannabis leaves, you can simply substitute kale or your favorite leafy greens to prepare this recipe at home.**

Tip! **This juice tastes "green," but it also has a hint of sweetness from the apple. If you'd like to add more sweetness, add a few slices of pineapple to the juicer, and then follow the recipe as directed.**

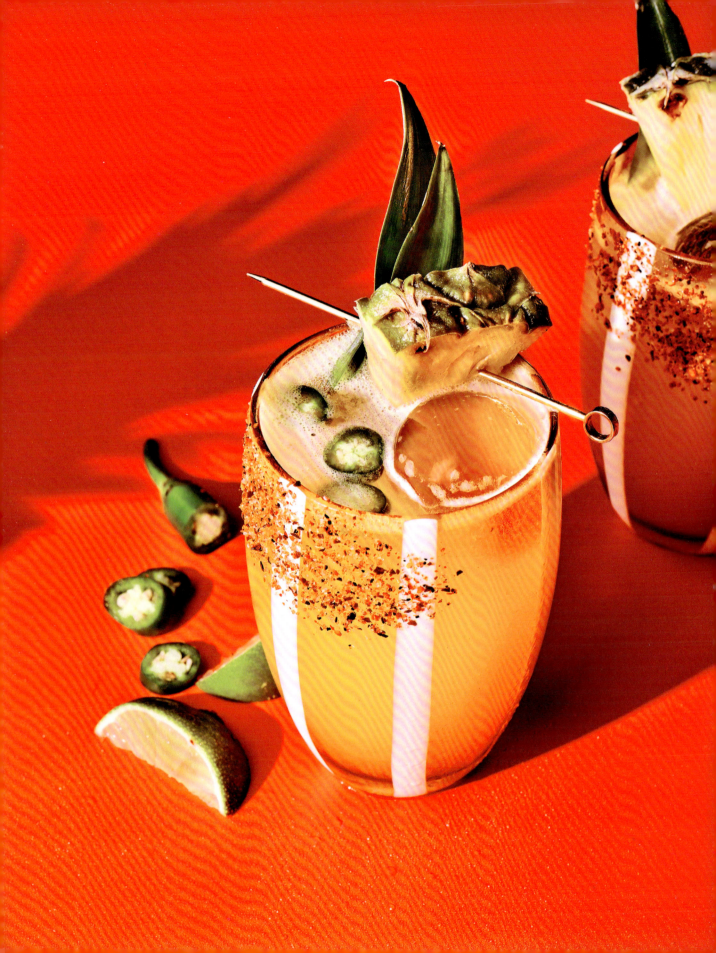

YIELD: 1 SERVING

SERRANO PINEAPPLE MARGARITA

For those who love spicy cocktails, this serrano pineapple margarita certainly brings the heat! For the best serrano flavor, the more efficient way to extract the pepper notes is to infuse the serrano into the tequila (see the instructions below). If serrano peppers are too spicy for your palate, feel free to swap for jalapeños, which add more mild spicy notes to this recipe. For those who love extremely spicy cocktails, instead of using serrano peppers, add habanero (if you're feeling brave!). Rim this cocktail with chile lime salt for extra flavor, and then enjoy.

+ TARGET DOSE:

5 to 10 mg THC | < 1 to 1 mg CBD per drink (using Cannabis-Infused Alcohol Tincture, page 58) or your preferred dose (using a commercially made THC tincture of your choice)

+ EQUIPMENT:

Saucer

Citrus juicer

Lowball glass

Shaker tin

Jigger

Hawthorne strainer

+ INGREDIENTS:

1 tablespoon chile lime salt (Tajín works great)

Lime wedge

3 ounces (90 mL) pineapple juice (see Resources on page 169)

2¼ ounces (67.5 mL) freshly squeezed lime juice

1 ounce (30 mL) serrano-infused tequila blanco (see to the right)

½ ounce (15 mL) triple sec

1 to 2 mL or your preferred dose Cannabis-Infused Alcohol Tincture (page 58)

Cubed ice

Pineapple leaf, 3 serrano rounds, and a slice of pineapple, for garnish

1. Add the chile lime salt to a shallow saucer. Rim the glass with a lime wedge, and then dip the glass into the salt to create a salted rim. Set aside.
2. To make the margarita, add the pineapple juice, lime juice, serrano-infused tequila, triple sec, and Cannabis-Infused Alcohol Tincture into a shaker tin. Add ice, cover, and then shake for 15 seconds or until cold.
3. Strain into a lowball glass filled with fresh ice. Garnish with a pineapple leaf, serrano rounds, and a slice of pineapple.

How to Make Serrano-Infused Tequila

When making a spicy margarita, one of the best techniques to capture the heat is to infuse hot peppers into the alcohol. Any hot pepper works, but for the purposes of this recipe, we use serrano peppers. If the serrano peppers are too spicy for your personal preference, simply swap for jalapeños.

1. To prepare this at home, simply cut 2 large serrano peppers into rounds, and combine with 1½ cups tequila blanco (or tequila of your choice) in a 16-ounce (480 mL) sterilized mason jar.
2. Shake to combine, and let the mixture rest for 24 hours.
3. Once ready, strain the solids from the liquids, and voilá! You've created a spicy serrano-infused tequila!

YIELD: 1 SERVING

SHISO MOJITO

During the peak of summer, there's nothing more refreshing than a mojito. This thirst-quenching cocktail can be made in a number of ways, but to add some unique flair, we love mixing in shiso to enhance the flavor. As a perfect aperitif or poolside sipper, this crisp canna-cocktail is infused with cannabis mint simple syrup, which compliments the shiso notes. By using simple syrup (instead of sugar, as some mixologists prefer), the ingredients in the drink blend more effortlessly, creating a well-balanced canna-cocktail.

+ TARGET DOSE:

5 to 10 mg THC | < 1 mg CBD per drink (using the Cannabis-Infused Mint Simple Syrup, page 61) or your preferred dose (using a commercially made THC alcohol tincture of your choice—see the below note)

+ EQUIPMENT:

Highball glass

Muddler

Bar spoon

+ INGREDIENTS:

1¼ ounces (38 mL) freshly squeezed lime juice

5 fresh shiso leaves

5 fresh mint leaves

¾ ounce (22 mL) Cannabis-Infused Mint Simple Syrup (page 61)

Cracked ice

1½ ounces (45 mL) white rum

Club soda

Fresh shiso leaf and a lime wedge, for garnish

1. Add the lime juice to the bottom of a highball glass.
2. Smack the shiso and mint leaves in your hand, and then add them to the bottom of the glass.
3. Using a muddler, gently muddle the ingredients to release the shiso and mint flavors.
4. Add the Cannabis-Infused Mint Simple Syrup, and then muddle again (be careful not to overmuddle and tear the leaves!).
5. Fill the glass to the top with cracked ice; then add the rum.
6. Top with club soda, stir to combine, and garnish with a fresh shiso leaf and a lime wedge before serving.

> *Tip!* If you don't have time to infuse the mint simple syrup with cannabis, you can still prepare this recipe by incorporating an alcohol-based tincture of your choice. Simply add it (at your preferred dose) during Step 3 to best integrate with the other ingredients, then follow the directions as noted.

YIELD: 1 SERVING

WATERMELON MINT LEMONADE

During peak watermelon season, we love making drinks using fresh watermelon juice, particularly cannabis-infused Watermelon Mint Lemonade! This refreshing nonalcoholic drink is incredibly easy to prepare and pairs well with just about any summer occasion. By combining watermelon, mint, and citrus flavors, this recipe quenches the thirst and serves as a perfect tart/sweet aperitif during cocktail hour for those who want an alcohol-free option. Because watermelon juice and lemonade run on the sweeter side, we love adding freshly squeezed lemon juice to brighten up the flavor and provide balance. The lemon juice can be adjusted up or down depending on your taste preferences. If you're a fan of salty/sweet combinations, be sure to add the chile salt rim for an extra kick of flavor!

+ TARGET DOSE:

5 to 10 mg THC | < 1 mg CBD per drink (using the Cannabis-Infused Mint Simple Syrup, page 61) or your preferred dose (using a commercially made THC tincture of your choice)

+ EQUIPMENT:

Blender or food processor

Fine-mesh strainer

16-ounce mason jar

Highball glass

Shaker tin

> **Tip!** Lemonade sweetness levels can vary, so feel free to adjust the freshly squeezed lemon juice amount until you find your preferred balance of sweet/tart flavors. Flip to "Resources" for a peek at what lemonade we used.

+ INGREDIENTS:

For the watermelon juice:

½ small seedless watermelon (this yields about 1 cup, so save the extra juice for more drinks)

For the Watermelon Mint Lemonade:

Lemon wedge

1 tablespoon chile lime salt (or Tajín)

3 ounces (90 mL) watermelon juice, pulp removed

4 ounces (120 mL) your favorite lemonade (see Resources on page 169)

1½ ounces (45 mL) freshly squeezed lemon juice (adjust depending on the lemonade and watermelon sweetness)

½ ounce (15 mL) Cannabis-Infused Mint Simple Syrup (page 61)

Ice

Watermelon slice, lemon wheel, and mint sprig, to garnish

1. Cut the watermelon in half, and add the watermelon flesh to a blender or food processor. Purée for 1 minute or until the watermelon chunks turn into juice.

2. Using a fine-mesh strainer, separate the pulp from the juice over a 16-ounce mason jar (save the extra juice to make more drinks). Discard the pulp, and set aside the mason jar.

3. Rim a glass of your choice with a lemon wedge, and dip the top of the glass into the Tajín to create a salted rim. Set aside.

4. Add the rest of the ingredients to a shaker tin. Add ice, and then shake for 15 seconds or until very cold. Strain into the salted glass filled with freshly cubed ice. Garnish with a watermelon slice, a lemon wheel, and a mint sprig before serving.

YIELD: 1 SERVING | YIELD: 1 MINI SMASH BURGER

THE DANKEST OVER-THE-TOP KIMCHI BLOODY MARY

Big, bold, and over-the-top, this is by far the dankest kimchi Bloody Mary we've ever prepared! Packed with flavor, spice, and all the right fixings, this canna-cocktail acts more like a meal, so be sure you have a big appetite before you create this recipe. Incorporating such special ingredients such as kimchi brine, togarashi salt, cabbage kimchi, sriracha, and a mini slider (yes, you read that right!), this indulgent Bloody Mary is like no other and is best enjoyed when those munchies kick in!

+ TARGET DOSE:

5 to 10 mg THC | < 1 to 1 mg CBD per milliliter (using Cannabis-Infused Alcohol Tincture, page 58) or your preferred dose (using a commercially made THC tincture of your choice)

+ EQUIPMENT:

For the Bloody Mary:

Blender

Boston shaker

Highball glass

Cocktail pick

Reusable straw

For the Mini Smash Burger:

Burger press or large metal spatula

Cast iron skillet

+ INGREDIENTS:

For the kimchi hot sauce (should yield 2 ounces):

2 tablespoons kimchi cabbage

1 ounce (30 mL) lime juice

1 teaspoon kimchi brine

1½ tablespoons sriracha

For the kimchi Bloody Mary:

2 ounces (60 mL) Kimchi hot sauce

7 ounces (60 mL) tomato juice

1 ounce (30 mL) soju (optional)

1 to 2 mL (or your preferred dose) Cannabis-Infused Alcohol Tincture (page 58)

1 or 2 dashes Worcestershire sauce

2 teaspoons pepperoncini juice

1½ teaspoons freshly prepared horseradish

Dash of celery salt

Dash of black pepper

Ice

Mini Smash Burger (page 145), cabbage kimchi, celery, your favorite olives and pickled veggies, lime wedge, and a sprinkle of togarashi salt, for garnish

For the Mini Smash Burger:

Mini Hawaiian roll

1.5 ounces high-quality grass-fed ground beef

1 small sliced onion

1 teaspoon garlic aioli

1 teaspoon mustard

Cheddar cheese

2 pickle slices

* Recipe continued on page 145

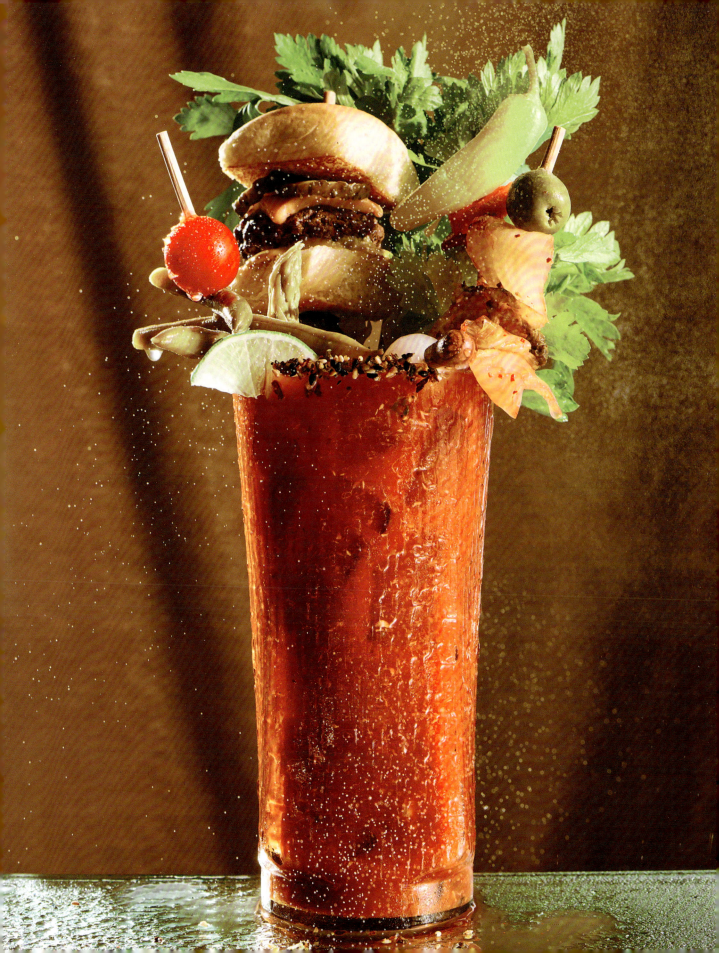

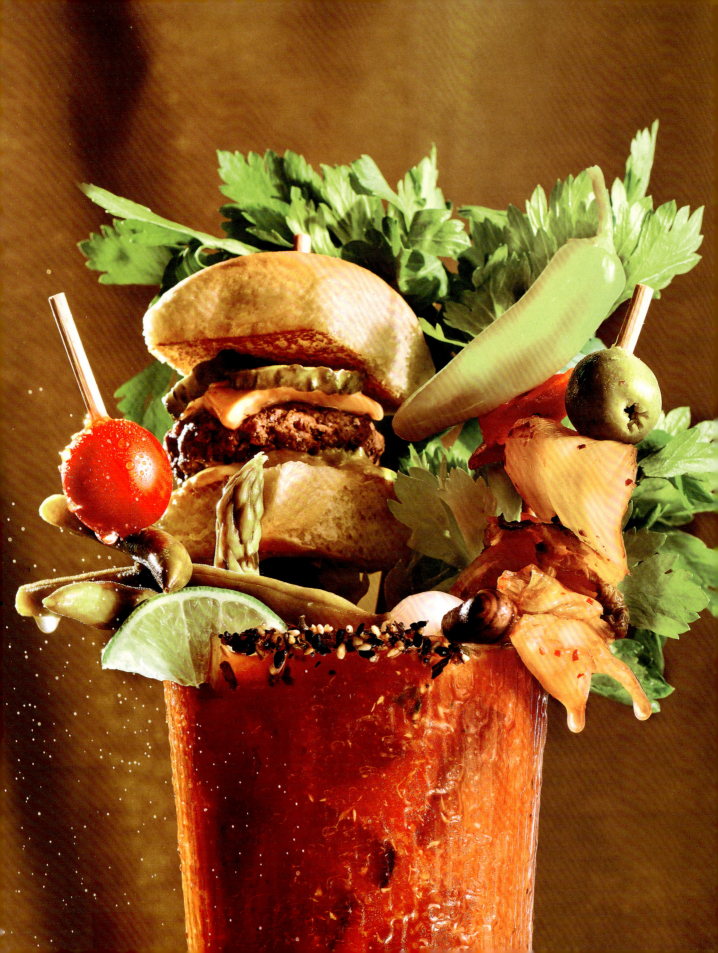

1. Begin by preparing the kimchi hot sauce. Add the kimchi cabbage, lime juice, kimchi brine, and sriracha to a single-serve blender. Blend on high until smooth, with no lumps remaining.
2. In a Boston shaker, empty the kimchi hot sauce into the bottom; then add the tomato juice, soju (if using), Cannabis-Infused Alcohol Tincture, Worcestershire sauce, pepperoncini juice, horseradish, celery salt, and black pepper in one part of the shaker.
3. To create the best Bloody Mary, you'll want to "roll" the liquid and ingredients together instead of shaking or stirring. To do so, fill a highball glass ¾ of the way with ice to accurately measure; then pour the ice into the other part of the Boston shaker. Pour the liquid ingredients over the ice, and then roll the liquid back and forth between both shakers about five or six times to mix the ingredients.
4. After mixing well, pour the liquid and ice into a highball glass. Garnish with a Mini Smash Burger (see below), cabbage kimchi, celery, olives, pickled veggies, a lime wedge, and togarashi salt sprinkled on top.
5. Serve immediately, and enjoy this over-the-top meal of a drink!

How to Make the Mini Smash Burger

We love a Bloody Mary with all the bells and whistles: pickles, olives, celery stick, bacon, shrimp cocktail, and even a mini slider. The more the merrier! Here's a recipe for a mini slider, the perfect over-the-top garnish for this drink that becomes a meal.

1. Weigh out beef, and shape into a ball.
2. Preheat a cast iron skillet over medium-high heat.
3. Place the ball of meat in the skillet, and smash it down into a thin patty with the press or a spatula. Season with salt and pepper. Cook for about 2 minutes.
4. Add some sliced onions on top, and flip the patty. Add a piece of cheese on top, and cook for another 2 to 3 minutes.
5. Cut the Hawaiian roll in half, and toast each side.
6. Assemble your mini burger. Smear mustard on the roll, add the patty, place pickles on top of the patty, smear the aioli on the other bun, and top the burger.
7. Repeat to make more sliders.

NONINFUSED
MUNCHIES

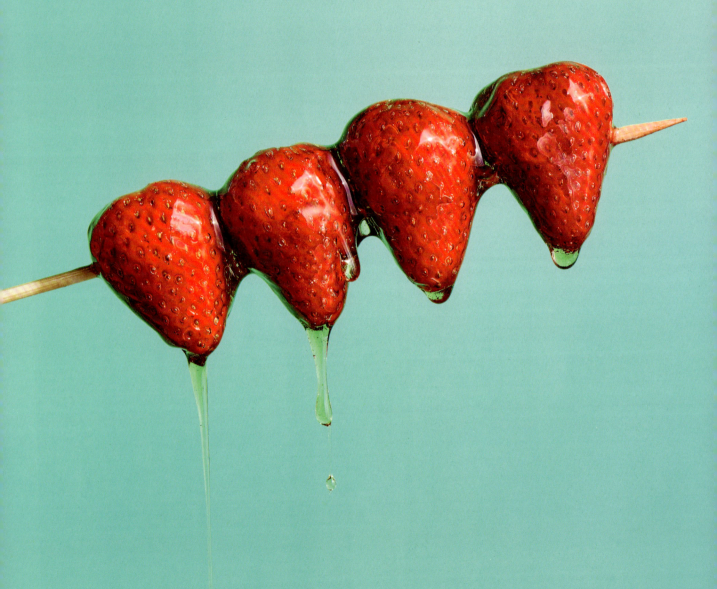

YIELD: 10 TO 15 SKEWERS

CANDIED FRUIT

Fruit is by far one of the best munchies! Sweet and juicy goes a long way for that cotton mouth. Most of us always have some sort of fruit lying around, so here's a fun and easy way to make fruit even more tempting—candied fruit! Whether you're using strawberries, tangerines, pineapple, or just about any other fruit, this easy-to-make recipe is quick and will satisfy your sweet tooth.

+ TARGET DOSE:

0 mg THC (*not* infused)

+ EQUIPMENT:

Saucepan

Skewers

Parchment paper

Thermometer

+ INGREDIENTS:

1 pound of fruit (strawberries, tangerines, pineapple, grapes, kiwi, or any other fruit you like)

2 cups granulated sugar

1 cup water

1. Skewer your fruit pieces, making sure they are completely dry.
2. In a medium saucepan, using a thermometer, bring the sugar and water to a boil until bubbling, at 300°F (149°C).
3. Dip the skewered fruit into the melted sugar, and spin to coat the fruit evenly.
4. Set the skewer on parchment paper, and let it harden (which should happen almost instantly).
5. Repeat steps 3 and 4 until all your fruit is used up or you run out of the sugar mixture.
6. Enjoy immediately; the fruit will weep and unharden the sugar over time.

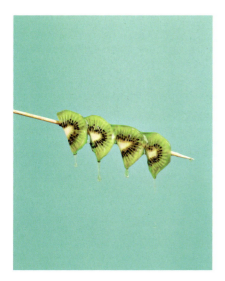
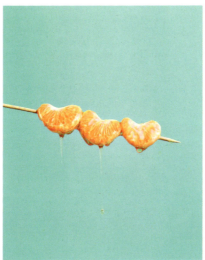
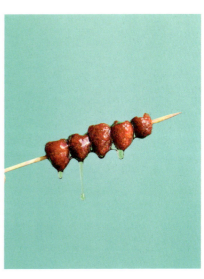

YIELD: ABOUT 20 TRUFFLES

CARROT CAKE TRUFFLES

RECIPE BY NICOLE DIMASCIO, CREATOR OF DOPE KITCHEN

FOLLOW ON INSTAGRAM @DOPE_KITCHEN

As a sweet, slightly-better-for-you treat, these carrot cake truffles are a deliciously compact and portable way to enjoy the taste of carrot cake in popable form. Made with white chocolate, carrots, almond butter, maple syrup, cream cheese filling, and so much more, these tasty truffles are the perfect option for dessert munchies.

TARGET DOSE:

0 mg THC per serving (*not* infused)

EQUIPMENT:

Piping bag

Parchment paper

Mini spatula

Medium mixing bowl

Food processor with grating attachment OR box grater

Measuring spoons

Measuring cups

Food scale, optional

INGREDIENTS:

For the cream cheese filling:

1 tablespoon butter, at room temperature

2 ounces cream cheese, at room temperature

¼ cup powdered sugar

For the truffles:

1 cup almond butter

2 tablespoons maple syrup

2 medium carrots, finely grated

½ teaspoon cinnamon

½ teaspoon nutmeg

½ teaspoon cloves

½ cup coconut flour

For the chocolate:

4 to 8 ounces white chocolate chips

2 teaspoons coconut oil

1. Mix together all the cream cheese filling ingredients, and drop about 24 pea-size dollops onto some parchment paper. Put the cream cheese drops in the freezer for about an hour.

2. Mix together all the truffle ingredients in a bowl. Using a tablespoon, scoop out 1 tablespoon of the mixture at a time onto a clean working surface. Flatten the small ball, and make a well in the center. Place a cream cheese filling dollop in the center; then carefully fold the cake mixture over the cream cheese, and roll it into a ball.

3. Set the truffle balls on a parchment-lined plate or baking sheet, and continue making balls until all the truffle mixture is used. Place the truffles in the freezer for 20 to 30 minutes.

4. Melt the white chocolate chips in the microwave or in a double boiler, and add the coconut oil. Stir until smooth.

5. Remove the truffles from the freezer, and coat each ball with chocolate. Let the excess chocolate drip off; then set the truffles on a parchment-lined dish or baking sheet.

6. Place the truffles back in the freezer for 20 minutes. Enjoy!

Tip! **You can replace the almond butter with another nut butter, if desired. We like cashew butter for its mild taste, allowing the other ingredients to shine. Peanut butter is a bit overpowering in flavor and is often too salty. The almond butter I used was very thick. If you use a loose/runny almond butter, you might need to use more coconut flour to absorb some of the moisture: Add about 1 tablespoon of coconut flour at a time until a thick consistency is achieved.**

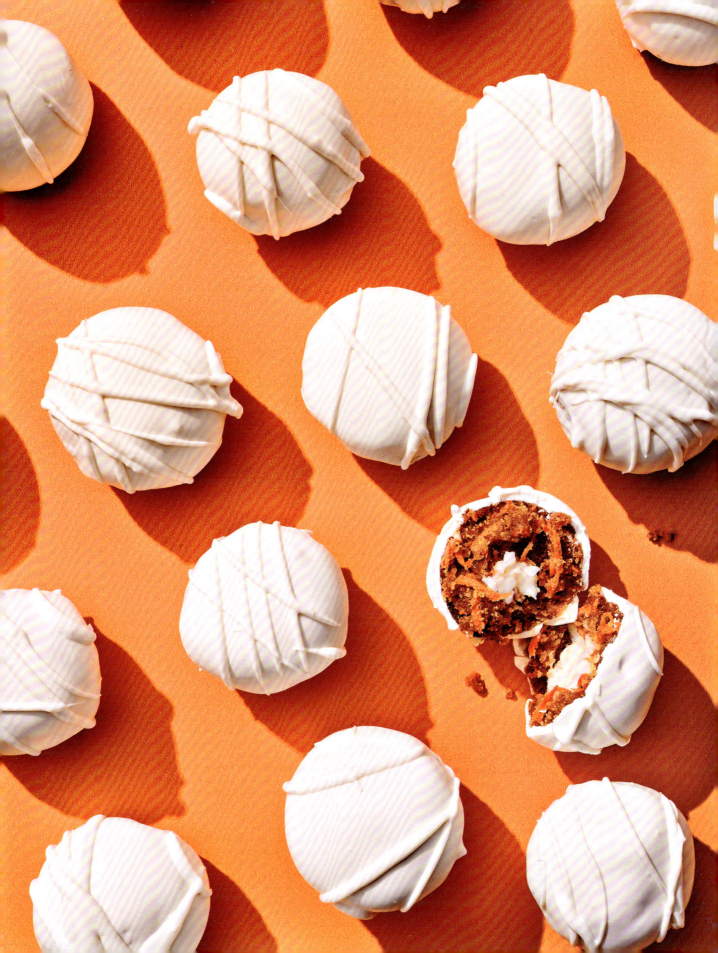

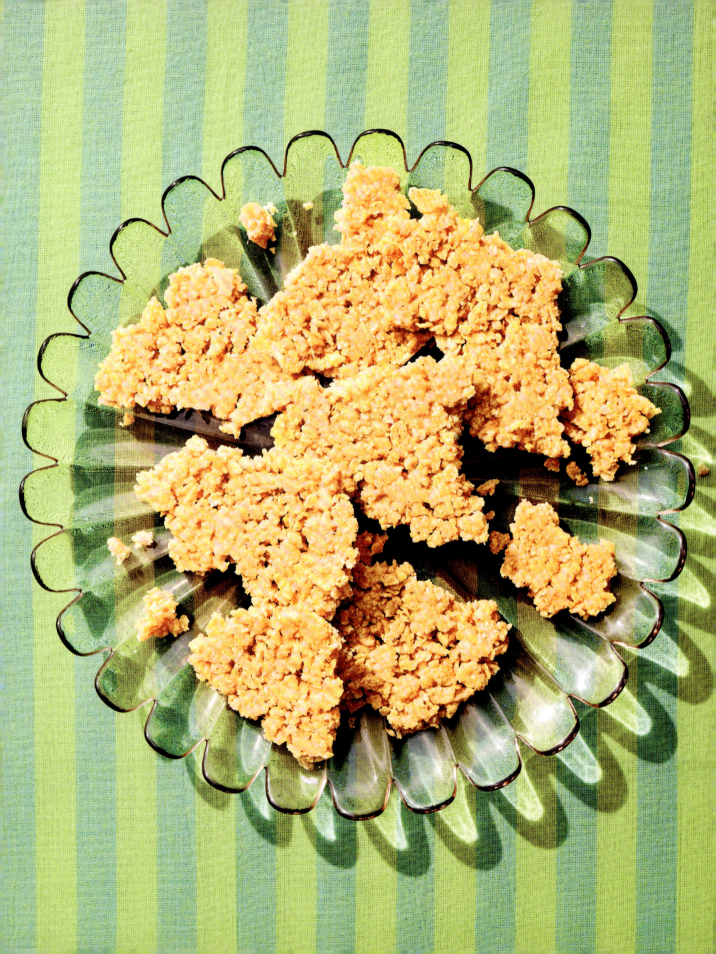

YIELD: 2 HALF-SHEET TRAYS, ABOUT 15 SERVINGS

CORNFLAKE MISO PRESSÉ

RECIPE BY VINCE BUGTONG, EXECUTIVE PASTRY CHEF & JAMES BEARD AWARD NOMINEE
FOLLOW ON INSTAGRAM @VINGOUGH

When preparing this recipe at home, the technique to make this snack is literally combining all the ingredients, pressing down the mixture, and rolling it out into a thin bark. Cornflakes have a crunchy texture but not much flavor. However, cornflakes can *absorb* the flavor from what they're mixed with. Almost resembling the taste and texture of cookies and cream, this unique combination adds umami from the miso and creamy decadence from the white chocolate.

TARGET DOSE:

0 mg THC (*not* infused)

EQUIPMENT:

Scale
Saucepan
Stainless steel bowl
Rubber spatula
Parchment paper
Rolling pin
Sheet pan

INGREDIENTS:

½ cup white chocolate
2 tablespoons brown butter
1 tablespoon shiro miso
3 cups cornflakes
⅛ teaspoon kosher salt

1. In a medium bowl, combine the white chocolate, brown butter, and miso. Melt this mixture over a double boiler. Stir until the mixture is homogeneous.
2. While waiting for the chocolate to melt, combine the cornflakes and salt into a separate bowl.
3. Crush the cornflakes into tiny uniform crumbs. Then pour the cornflakes over the chocolate. Fold the mixture until the cereal is completely coated.
4. Pour the cereal mixture onto some parchment paper, and then place another piece of parchment over the mixture.
5. Using a rolling pin, roll the mixture in the parchment paper slowly and gently so that the bark stays in one piece.
6. When the Cornflake Miso Pressé is evenly rolled out, place it onto a sheet pan and freeze for at least 2 hours.
7. When ready, you can break the bark into your desired sizes. Store in an airtight container, and keep frozen.

Tip! You can use any chocolate for this recipe, but couverture chocolate is recommended for the most high-quality product.

YIELD: 4 SERVINGS

RECIPE BY MENNLAY GOLOKEH AGGREY, AUTHOR OF *THE ART OF WEED BUTTER*
FOLLOW ON INSTAGRAM @MENNLAY

FRIED CASSAVA FRIES

In Ghana, almost every farming family has a cassava patch growing around the farm. Cassava (a.k.a. agbeli, yuca, and manioc) is a prehistoric plant native to the southern region of the Brazilian Amazon and is known as one of the most popular, most integral food staples in West Africa, South America, Thailand, and the Caribbean. These drought-resistant, starchy, protein-packed root vegetables also contain vitamin C and hella fiber, making them a much better alternative to french fries. Consider these the ultimate snack for when munchies attack. Dip in a green sauce (see below) or aioli, or eat them as is. They're that good.

EQUIPMENT:

- Large pot
- Skillet
- Bamboo skimmer

INGREDIENTS:

- 2 to 4 cassavas
- 16 ounces coconut, grapeseed, or canola oil (for frying)
- Pinch of flaky salt
- 1 teaspoon smoked paprika (optional)
- Pinch of chopped cilantro, to garnish (optional)

Spicy Green Dipping Sauce

EQUIPMENT:

- Food processor

INGREDIENTS:

- 2 ripe avocados, peeled, pitted, and scooped
- 1 head garlic, peeled, crushed, and finely chopped
- 1 small white or sweet onion, minced
- 2 limes, juiced
- 1 jalapeño, finely diced
- Pinch of coarse salt
- 1 bunch cilantro, chopped

1. Using a sharp knife, carefully cut the cassava, removing all the skin. (Don't bother using a vegetable peeler: It's not efficient and might not safely remove all the skin.) Then cut the cassava into large pieces.

2. In a large pot, bring water to a boil over medium heat; add the peeled cassava chunks to the water. Boil until the cassava is fork tender, about 30 minutes. Turn off the burner, and let cool.

3. Once cooled, remove the root core in the center of the cassava, pat dry, and cut the cassava into the size and shape of thick steak fries.

4. Add oil to a large skillet. Heat on medium-high for 30 to 60 seconds until you see tiny air bubbles start to form. Gently place the cassava in the skillet, and fry, turning over all sides until golden brown.

5. When the cassava is fried to your desired crispiness, use a skimmer to remove the fries to a plate lined with wax paper or a paper towel, to remove excess oil.

6. Place the cassava fries in a dish, and dust with flaky salt and cayenne. If desired, top with chopped cilantro.

> *Tip!* Cassava is known to be toxic if it is eaten raw, but it's rare that anyone gets sick from eating it raw. Please do use caution, however, and make sure that the cassava is cooked thoroughly.

Spicy Green Dipping Sauce

This delicious dip can be paired with the cassava fries or literally any other dish that needs a kick.

1. In a large bowl, add all the ingredients. Mix with a fork until it reaches a thin but not watery consistency. If preferred, use a food processor on a low pulse until all ingredients are creamy yet chunky.

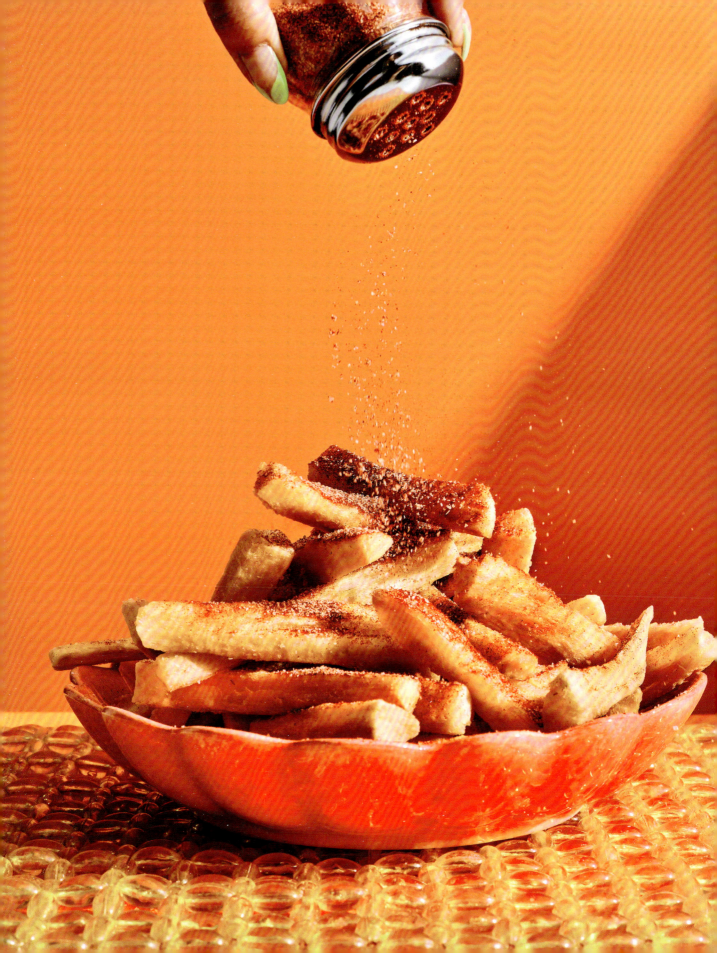

YIELD: 4 GRILLED CHEESE SANDWICHES

GRILLED CHEESE WITH CARAMELIZED ONIONS

Grilled cheese and caramelized onions—a stoner's dream come true! Who doesn't love an elevated grilled cheese, especially when you have the munchies? There's nothing better than the perfect handheld cheese-pull moment. When preparing this recipe, you'll quickly notice that the umami from the caramelized onions is a game changer, so don't skip this step. Although it does take some time, it's worth every bite. Trust us, you'll want seconds!

+ TARGET DOSE:

0 mg THC (*not* infused)

+ EQUIPMENT:

Bread knife

Pan

Spatula

+ INGREDIENTS:

1 pound white onions, chopped into ¼-inch strips

2 tablespoon avocado oil, to coat the pan

Pinch of salt

Pinch of black pepper

1 tablespoon butter

1 loaf sourdough bread

Butter (enough to coat each side of the bread)

5 ounces aged white cheddar

5 ounces pepper jack cheese

1. Chop the onions into quarter-inch strips.
2. Add the onions to a large pan on medium-low heat, along with a little bit of avocado oil (about 2 tablespoons) to lightly coat. Stirring often, keep browning the onions until they are a rich caramelized brown and super soft, about 45 minutes. During the last 5 minutes, add a pinch of salt, a pinch of pepper, and 1 tablespoon butter. Set aside.
3. Using a serrated bread knife, cut the sourdough loaf into 1-inch slices.
4. Generously butter the outer side of 2 slices of bread.
5. Assemble your grilled cheese with one layer of caramelized onions, a slice or thin layer of white cheddar, and another slice or thin layer of pepper jack cheese.
6. On high heat, preheat a pan until it is pipping hot. Place one side of the assembled grilled cheese sandwich down on the pan. You should hear a sizzle. Immediately lower the heat to medium, and cook until crispy and golden brown. Check underneath with a spatula to make sure it is perfectly crispy, about 2 minutes.
7. Flip, and repeat for each sandwich.

Tip! To maintain the crispy, crunchy texture of the grilled cheese, when pulling it off the pan, be sure to move your grilled cheese to a wire rack (so it doesn't steam on itself) until you're ready to serve (especially when working in batches). You can also pop it back in the oven at 350°F for a couple minutes to warm it back up, but it is best enjoyed immediately. Also, the better the bread, the better the grilled cheese, so try to get the best sourdough loaf you can find.

YIELD: 12 TO 15 MINI CORN DOGS

MINI KOREAN CORN DOGS

Is it still a corn dog if there's no cornmeal in the batter? We think so! This cult-classic American staple is all the rave on the streets of Seoul as one of the most beloved street foods. The main difference between American corn dogs and Korean dogs is the batter: no cornmeal. Instead, it's a glutinous rice flour mixture. Korean corn dogs also come with an array of wild toppings (such as corn dogs covered in French fries) and non–hot dog fillings (such as fishcake and cheese). This is our version, and it's truly one of our favorite munchies to indulge in. Enjoy!

+ TARGET DOSE:

0 mg THC (*not* infused)

+ EQUIPMENT:

Mixing bowl
Measuring spoons
Wire rack
Wok or large pot

+ INGREDIENTS:

4 to 5 mozzarella cheese sticks or pepper jack cheese sticks, cut in thirds

Uncured cocktail beef frankfurters

For the batter:

½ cup all-purpose flour
1 cup glutinous rice flour
1 tablespoon sugar
½ teaspoon baking powder
¼ teaspoon salt
1 egg
1 cup cold water
Panko breadcrumbs
Vegetable oil, for frying

1. In a medium mixing bowl, combine the all-purpose flour, glutinous rice flour, sugar, baking powder, and salt.
2. Add the egg and cold water, and whisk until smooth.
3. Pour the panko breadcrumbs into a shallow bowl or small tray.
4. Heat the vegetable oil in a pot or wok between 350°F and 375°F (176°C and 190°C).
5. Dip the beef frankfurters and cheese sticks into the batter one at a time until they're fully coated. Then roll into the panko breadcrumbs.
6. Carefully drop the coated mini corn dogs into the hot oil, and fry for about 3 to 4 minutes until they're crispy and golden brown.
7. Remove the corn dogs from the oil, and place on a wire rack lined with paper towels to remove excess grease.
8. Serve hot with your choice of dipping sauce: ketchup, ranch, honey mustard, sriracha mayo, or all of the above! The street vendors in Korea also dust extra sugar on their corn dogs (but this is optional).

YIELD: 4 SERVINGS

SALVADORAN PUPUSAS

RECIPE BY MANNY MENDOZA, CHEF AND CREATOR OF HERBAL NOTES
FOLLOW ON INSTAGRAM @MANOFROM18TH

This is a meaningful recipe to me because the pupusa is the main staple dish of the tiny country of El Salvador, where my family is from. I also demonstrate a version of these pupusas on the Netflix show *Cooked with Cannabis*, Episode 6. Pupusas are an art form that require some time and practice to master the most delicately perfect consistency. They're easy but not exactly simple. But for a stoner cook such as myself, I find much comfort and meditation in preparing pupusas while baking myself—not to mention the extreme satisfaction of enjoying a cheesy, hot, and toasty end product. I always tell people that the best pupusa with all the right fixings is better than any slice of pizza anywhere.

+ TARGET DOSE:
0 mg THC (*not* infused)

+ EQUIPMENT:
Measuring cups
Kitchen scale
Mixing bowl (or stand mixer)
Wooden spoon
Cheese grater
Cast iron pan, or any flat griddle
Spatula

+ INGREDIENTS:

For the masa dough:
1 pound corn flour (masa harina or maseca)
2 teaspoons salt
1 tablespoon chicken or veggie bouillon
2 ounces margarine
2 cups water, simmering hot
1¼ cups cold water
1 cup grated cheese
½ cup cotija cheese

For the potato, squash, and cheese filling:
1 teaspoon ground cumin
1 teaspoon oregano
1 teaspoon garlic powder
2 teaspoons salt
3 potatoes, peeled and boiled to tender
3 Mexican squash, grated
1½ pounds chihuahua and/or mozzarella cheese

Recipe continued on page 159

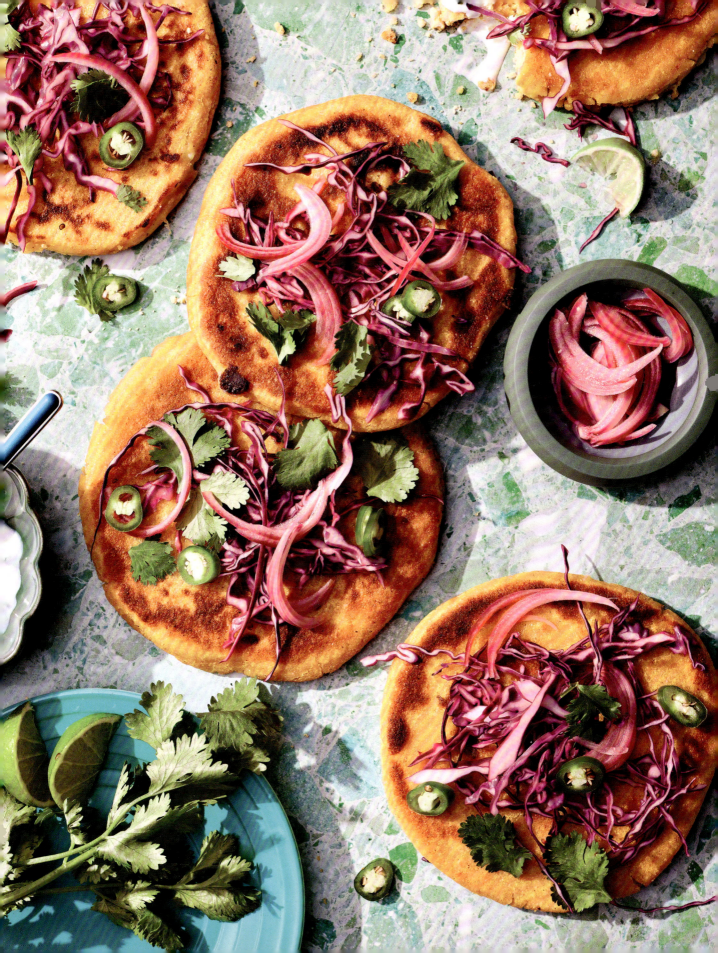

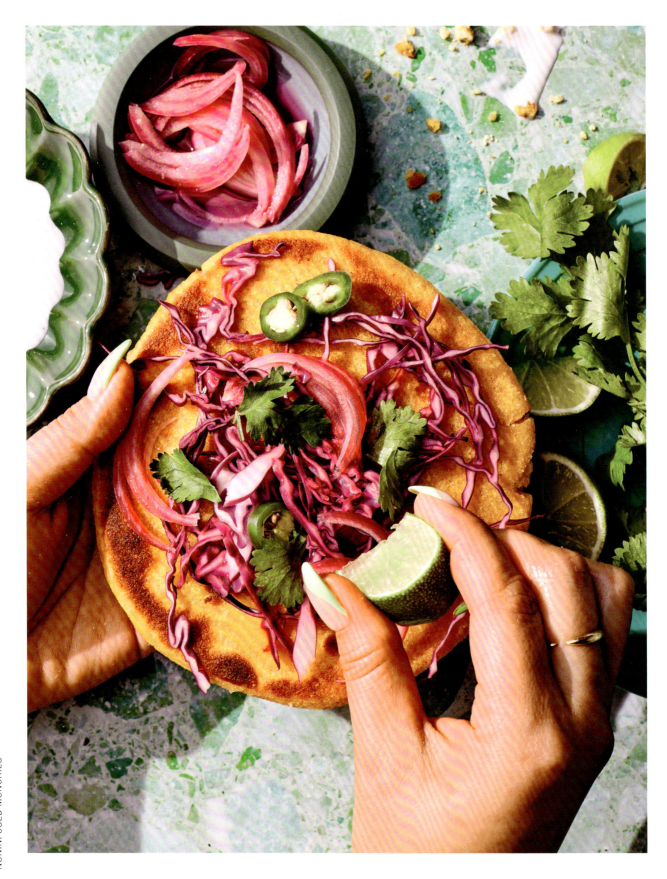

1. Combine the flour, salt, bouillon, and margarine in a medium mixing bowl.

2. Add the hot water to the flour mixture, and stir with a wooden spoon until thoroughly combined.

3. Once combined, add the cold water, and begin to mix with your hands. Work thoroughly for 10 minutes until the dough becomes soft and pliable. If the dough feels too dry, add some water; if it feels too wet, add some corn flour until you feel a soft dough that isn't sticky but also isn't dry. You can use a stand mixer for faster results, although working the dough by hand is crucial to developing a feel for the right consistency.

4. Set aside a small bowl of water combined with 1 tablespoon of any cooking oil.

5. For the filling, combine the seasonings from the ingredients list along with the cooked potatoes, grated squash, and cheese in a mixing bowl. Mix with a spoon until everything is thoroughly combined into a smooth mixture.

6. Set up your pupusa-making station: the dough mixture in a bowl, the veggie/cheese filling, and a small bowl of water/oil.

7. Before you start the pupusas, grease your cast iron pan and preheat to medium heat.

8. Take about a 6-ounce ball of dough in your hands, compact it in a circular motion, and then slightly flatten it into a puck shape. At this point, use your opposite hand to make a closed fist, and press your fist into the dough to make a cavity where you will insert the filling. Make as deep a cavity as possible without breaking the dough.

9. Once you have a cavity in your dough, add enough filling (don't be too stingy) to each dough ball, but make sure that the filling isn't overflowing. Find a happy medium of filling that feels workable for you.

10. Once filled, enclose your dough package using both hands in a twisting/sealing motion. This takes a little practice, but in no time, you will be a pro at this. Once sealed, if there's any extra dough, remove it so that your pupusa isn't too doughy.

11. When your pupusa ball is filled and sealed, lightly wet your hands in the water/oil mixture to keep your pupusa from sticking. Flatten your pupusa with both hands in clapping motion, making sure the edges are smooth and not cracking. You want a happy medium of not too thick and not too thin of a pupusa. When you're ready, add the pupusa to the griddle. You should hear a gentle sizzle, not an aggressive one; cook about 4 to 5 minutes on each side. Continue making pupusas while you are cooking them simultaneously.

> *Tip!* **Serve with lightly pickled cabbage, an infused salsa, or a condiment of your choice. You can never go wrong with Salvadoran crema from your local Latin grocery store. If you're feeling like a fungi and you want even more vegetarian deliciousness, add some chopped roasted mushrooms to your veggie mixture, for extra umami.**

YIELD: 4 SERVINGS

SICHUAN TOOTHPICK LAMB

> RECIPE BY WENDY ZENG, CHEF AND DISCOVERY PLUS "CHOPPED 420" WINNER
> FOLLOW ON INSTAGRAM @WENYERHUNGRY

When hosting a party, this munchie snack is going to be your best friend! Savory and delicious, this recipe combines bite-size crispy lamb seasoned with Sichuan's iconic mala spice. It's served with a toothpick, so it's ideal if you're hosting guests because it's so easy to share. Made with a variety of Asian spices, this perfectly seasoned lamb appetizer will keep you salivating.

+ TARGET DOSE:

0 mg THC (*not* infused)

+ EQUIPMENT:

Small pan
Large wok or deep frying pan
Spider/slotted ladle
Spice grinder
Prep/mixing bowls
Toothpicks

+ INGREDIENTS:

½ cinnamon stick
1 star anise pod
2 teaspoons Sichuan peppercorn (½ for frying), divided
1 tablespoon cumin seeds (⅓ for frying), divided
1-pound boneless lamb shoulder/leg
1 tablespoon soy sauce
1 tablespoon rice wine
¼ teaspoon baking soda
½ teaspoon white pepper
1 teaspoon grated ginger
⅓ cup dried red chili pods
2 cups canola/vegetable oil
4 cloves garlic, minced
½ tablespoon toasted sesame seeds
1½ cups cilantro

1. Break up the cinnamon stick and star anise, and place in a small pan with 1 teaspoon of the Sichuan peppercorn and ⅔ tablespoon cumin seeds. Toast the spices on low heat until aromatics release and the spices are looking slightly brown and toasty. Swirl the pan often to keep the spices toasting evenly.
2. Transfer the toasted spices to a spice grinder, and grind until fine. Set aside the spice mixture.
3. Cutting against the grain, slice the lamb into slices ½ inch thick by 2 inches long. Marinate with the soy sauce, rice wine, baking soda, white pepper, ginger, and the reserved ground spice mix. Let the lamb marinate for at least 1 hour.
4. Soak the toothpicks in a bowl filled with water for at least 30 minutes.
5. Meanwhile, cut the dried chili pods in half, and put them in a bowl with the remaining whole Sichuan peppercorn and cumin seeds so that this is ready to go in the wok later.
6. Roughly chop the cilantro into 2-inch sticks, keeping as much of the stem as possible.
7. Skewer each lamb piece on a toothpick. Heat 2 cups oil in a wok or deep sauté pan. Deep-fry the tooth-picked lamb pieces in batches, so as not to crowd them. Be sure you don't lower the temperature of the oil too drastically.
8. When the lamb is browned and crispy around the edges, remove the pieces with a slotted ladle onto a plate lined with two layers of paper towels.
9. Strain the oil to discard any leftover fried bits, and add about 3 tablespoons of oil in the wok/pan. Heat to medium high, and cook the garlic and dried chili spice mixture. Once the garlic is fragrant and the color begins to change, dump all the fried lamb pieces back in, to sauté together.
10. Taste and add salt, if needed. Turn off the heat, garnish with some extra cilantro, sesame seeds, and serve.

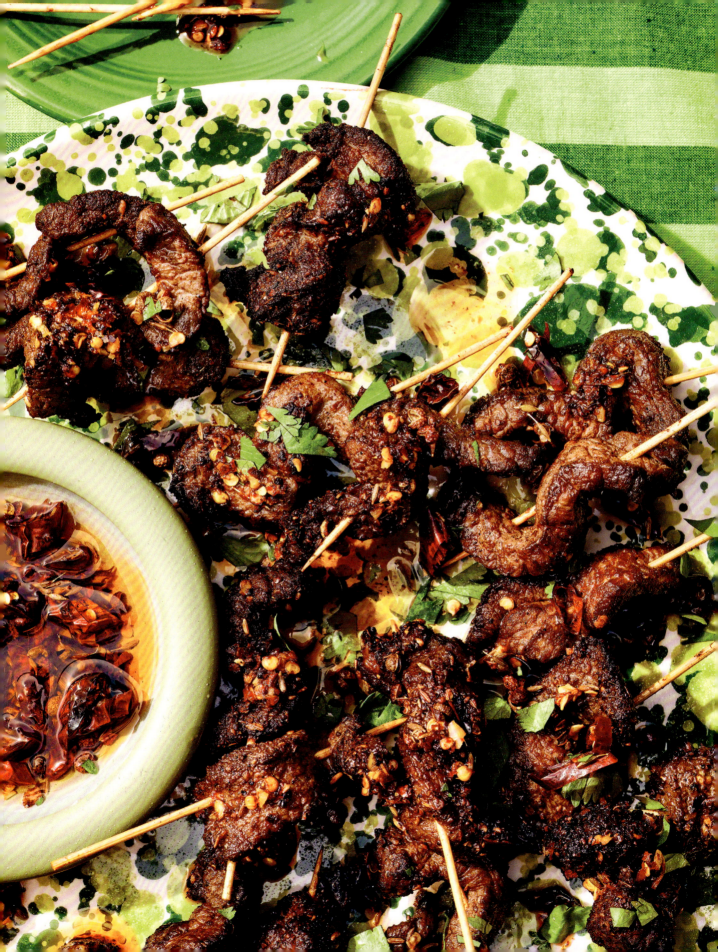

YIELD: 4 TO 5 SERVINGS

CANDIED SWEET POTATOES

During the holiday season or anytime you're in the mood for a delicious serving of candied sweet potatoes, be sure to bookmark this recipe! Baked until golden brown and covered in black sesame seeds, this tasty dish is a staple when it comes to comfort food. For our take on this classic side dish, we used Korean or Japanese sweet potatoes, which have a sweeter taste and a nuttier flavor than ordinary sweet potato varieties.

+ TARGET DOSE:

0 mg THC (*not* infused)

+ EQUIPMENT:

Pot for frying

Nonstick saucepan

Parchment paper

Measuring spoons

+ INGREDIENTS:

Oil for deep frying (depending on size of pot)

2 pounds Korean or Japanese Sweet Potatoes, chopped into 2-inch pieces

Pinch of salt

3 tablespoons avocado oil

1 cup sugar

1 tablespoon black sesame seeds

1. Add enough oil to a pot to fry sweet potatoes, about 2½ inches. Using a thermometer, bring the oil to 350°F (176°C).
2. Add the sweet potatoes to the pan, and deep-fry until they're golden brown and cooked through. Be careful not overcrowd the pot, and work in batches, if necessary.
3. Transfer the sweet potatoes to a wire rack, and season with salt.
4. Prepare a plate with parchment paper. Set aside.
5. In a nonstick saucepan, add the avocado oil on low heat, and then add the sugar. Do not stir yet.
6. Wait for the sugar to start melting and turn into a light syrup. Then slowly swirl the syrup in the pan, to avoid burning. Timing is crucial; it can burn quickly!
7. When the sugar is a golden caramel color and bubbling and/or foaming, add the sweet potatoes, and quickly toss together so that each piece is coated evenly.
8. Transfer the potatoes onto your parchment-lined plate, spreading them apart so they don't all stick together. Sprinkle with black sesame before they harden.
9. Enjoy immediately; the hard candied shell will become soggy over time.

YIELD: EIGHT TO TEN 3-OUNCE POPSICLES

CHOCOLATE MILK TEA POPSICLE

This chocolatey popsicle dessert is beyond satisfying, especially when chocolate cravings hit! If you're unfamiliar with milk tea, it is absolutely one of our favorites, especially when combined with the rich, nutty decadence that is a hazelnut spread. Perfect to enjoy during a hot summer day (or, really, anytime you're wanting chocolate), this unique combination of flavors is a mouthwatering treat for any sweet tooth.

+ TARGET DOSE:

0 mg THC (*not* infused)

+ EQUIPMENT:

3-ounce popsicle mold

Popsicle sticks

Blender

+ INGREDIENTS:

40 grams (20 bags) Earl Grey tea to make 1 cup of brewed black tea

1¼ cups water

2 tablespoons condensed milk

1 cup half-and-half

Pinch of sea salt

½ cup chocolate hazelnut spread

1. Steep 40 grams or 20 bags of Earl Grey tea in 1¼ cups of 90°F (32°C) water. Any hotter, and the tea can become bitter. Let the tea steep for at least an hour.
2. Once cool, strain all the tea leaves, add condensed milk to the strained tea, and stir.
3. Add the milk tea to a blender with the half-and-half, salt, and chocolate hazelnut spread, and blend until smooth.
4. Pour into popsicle molds, leaving some space at the top because it will expand in the freezer.
5. Insert your popsicle sticks, and freeze for at least 3 to 4 hours. Then enjoy!

Tip! **If the popsicles are difficult to remove from the mold, run hot water on the outside of the mold for a few seconds, and gently pull them loose. This recipe does have a bit of caffeine from the tea, so be aware, especially if you're sensitive to caffeine and are indulging in a late-night snack.**

YIELD: 2 PAVLOVAS

STRAWBERRIES AND CREAM PAVLOVA

RECIPE BY MONICA LO, CREATOR OF SOUS WEED® AND AUTHOR OF *THE WEED GUMMIES COOKBOOK*
FOLLOW ON INSTAGRAM @SOUSWEED

True story: I delivered the manuscript for *The Weed Gummies Cookbook* the same week I delivered my son. These days, I'm making way more baby food than cannabis edibles. But mom and dad also deserve a treat, especially after a long day of toddler wrangling! I often make meringue cookies for my baby and use the rest of the egg whites to make airy pavlovas with a crisp exterior and a soft, pillowy center. This Strawberries and Cream Pavlova is a staple in our household because all the elements can be made ahead of time and quickly assembled. The combination of crisp meringue, luscious cream, juicy strawberries, and refreshing mint is truly divine!

+ EQUIPMENT:

Stand mixer or hand mixer with a whisk attachment

Silicone baking mat

+ INGREDIENTS:

For the pavlova:

3 egg whites, at room temperature

¾ cup superfine sugar

½ teaspoon vanilla extract

½ teaspoon cream of tartar

1 teaspoon cornstarch

For the topping:

1 cup cold heavy whipping cream

1 tablespoon superfine sugar

8 strawberries, halved

Mint, to garnish

Cannabis leaves, to garnish (optional)

> *Tip!* Even the smallest speck of egg yolk can render your pavlova flat and unusable, so be gentle when separating your whites from the yolk. Room-temperature egg whites will whip up to a greater volume, with an airier texture, than cold egg whites.

1. Preheat the oven to 300°F (149°C). Line a baking sheet with a silicone baking mat.

2. With a stand mixer or hand mixer fitted with a whisk attachment, beat the egg whites in a large, clean bowl on medium-high speed until soft peaks form.

3. Add the sugar in three additions, beating for 30 seconds in between. Once all the sugar has been added, turn up the mixer to high speed, and continue beating until stiff peaks form. Scrape down the sides of the bowl to make sure all the sugar has been incorporated. The mixture will be thick and shiny, and when you hold the whisk upright, the peaks won't budge.

4. Add the vanilla extract, cream of tartar, and cornstarch, and beat for 2 seconds on the lowest speed to incorporate. The peaks should still be very stiff.

5. Spoon the pavlova mixture into two 6-inch circles on a silicone baking mat. Give the pavlova some height by dolloping the mixture to make a tall pile. The edges should be higher, with a slight dip in the center.

6. Place the pavlovas in the oven, and immediately reduce the heat to 200°F (93°C). Bake for 1 hour and 15 minutes. Do not open the oven door at all during this time because the pavlovas may crack.

7. Turn off the oven, and do not open the door. Allow the pavlova to cool and dehydrate even more inside the oven for 2 to 3 hours.

8. With a stand mixer or hand mixer fitted with a whisk attachment, beat the heavy cream until it begins to thicken. Add sugar, and continue to beat until soft peaks form. The whipped cream should be thick and smooth; if it becomes grainy, it's overwhipped. Store in the refrigerator until it's time for assembly.

9. To assemble, place a pavlova shell on a serving dish, and add generous dollops of whipped cream across the center. Arrange strawberries on top, and garnish with mint and cannabis leaves.

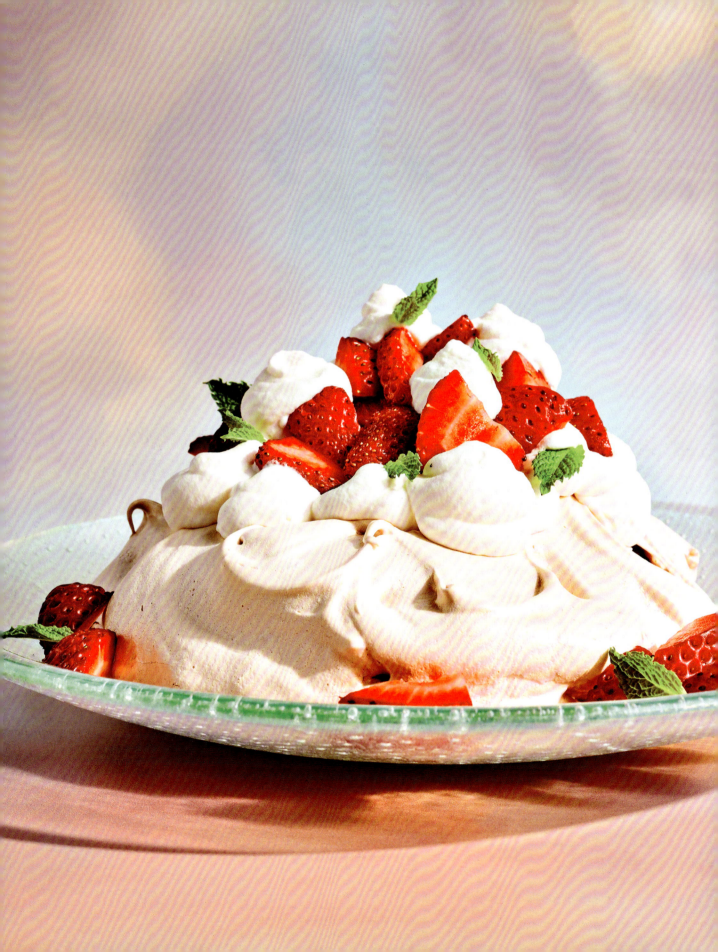

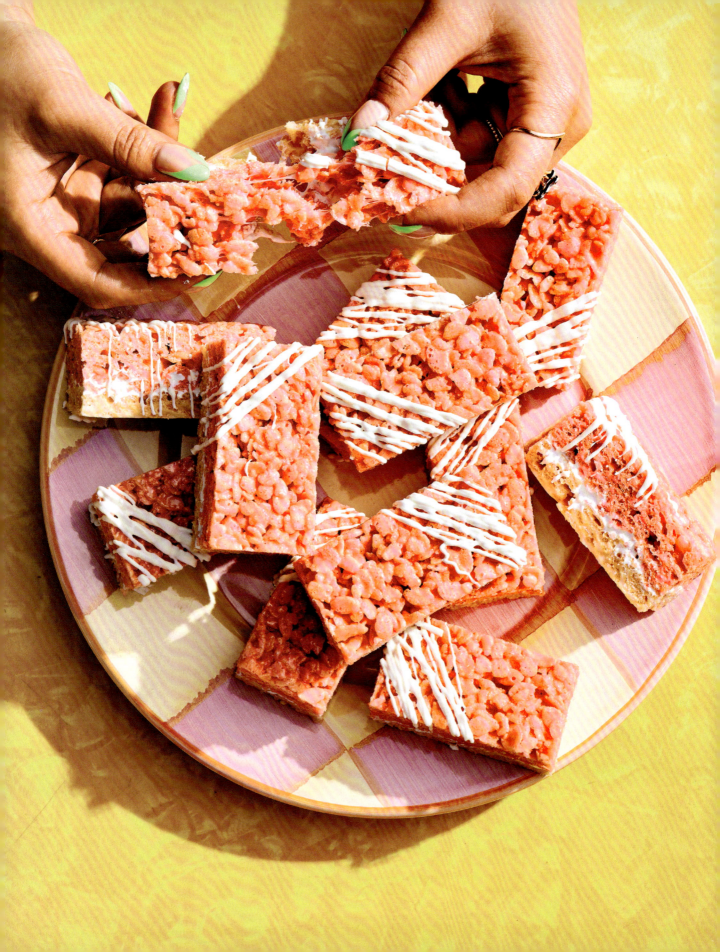

YIELD: 18 CRISPY RICE TREATS

STRAWBERRY WHITE RABBIT CRISPY RICE TREATS

RECIPE BY CHRISTOPHER JACOB, CREATOR OF THE HAWAIIAN ALCHEMIST

FOLLOW ON INSTAGRAM @THE.HAWAIIAN.ALCHEMIST

This recipe is a mashup of all things that made my childhood sweet and fun. It's a classic Asian candy combined with a nostalgic American treat, all in an overly complicated, elevated recipe. Have fun!

+ EQUIPMENT:

9-by-13-inch pan
4-quart pan
Flat rubber spatula
Foil
Brush
Large pot (7 quarts)

+ INGREDIENTS:

2 tablespoons water

2 tablespoons condensed cream

18 pieces White Rabbit candy, unwrapped (leave the transparent rice paper on)

1 cup unsalted butter, divided

Two 10-ounce bags (11 heaping cups) mini marshmallows, divided

½ teaspoon pure vanilla extract

Pinch of salt

9 cups crispy rice cereal, divided

4 ounces (½ a jar) marshmallow cream

½ teaspoon strawberry extract

6 drops pink food coloring

6 ounces white melting wafers or white compound chocolate

3 grams edible gold luster dust (optional)

1. In a small microwave-safe bowl, combine the water and condensed milk and the White Rabbit candies. Microwave on high for 20 seconds. Remove and stir. Return to the microwave at intervals for 5 seconds until the mixture melts completely. The texture should resemble a white caramel sauce.

2. Line a 9-by-13-inch baking pan with parchment paper. Lightly grease the parchment. (I always use a very light mist of nonstick spray.) Set aside.

3. Melt ¼ cup butter over medium heat in a large pot. Once melted, add 4 cups of marshmallows. Stir the mixture until the marshmallows are completely melted.

4. Remove from heat, and stir in the vanilla extract, salt, and White Rabbit mixture. Mix well until combined. Fold in 3 cups of cereal. Make sure each piece of cereal is coated with the marshmallow mixture.

5. Transfer the mixture to the prepared pan. Using a lightly greased rubber spatula, gently spread the mixture to fit the pan. Do not pack it down; just press down so that it's secure in the pan, flush with the corners, and leveled in the pan.

6. Let the mixture cool, and allow to set for at least 1 hour (and up to 1 day) at room temperature. Cover tightly if you'll be leaving it out for more than a few hours.

7. Spread the marshmallow cream evenly over the top of the cereal.

8. Melt the remaining butter over medium heat in a very large pot. Once melted, add the remaining marshmallows. Stir until the marshmallows are completely melted.

9. Remove from heat, and stir in the strawberry extract and 6 drops of pink food coloring. Fold in the remaining cereal.

10. Transfer the mixture to the top of the pan with the White Rabbit and marshmallow cream layer. Using a lightly greased spatula, very gently press the mixture into the pan so that it's secure in the pan, making enough contact with the marshmallow layer, and is evenly distributed and level.

11. Let the mixture cool for an hour. (If you're in a rush, you can place the pan in the fridge for about 10 minutes.)

Recipe continued on page 168

12. Lift the cereal treats out as one giant piece from the pan, using the parchment paper. Cut into 3-by-1½-inch squares.

13. Place the white chocolate melting wafers into a microwave-safe bowl, and microwave for 10 seconds; remove and stir. Place the bowl back in the microwave for 10 seconds; remove and stir. If the chocolate isn't melted completely (it's smooth and runny), return the bowl to the microwave for intervals of 5 seconds, removing and stirring until all pieces are melted.

14. Using a ½ tablespoon, dollop the melted chocolate onto the center of each cereal piece, "swoosh" it around with the back of the spoon, or just drizzle across each crispy rice cereal treat. Get creative—you've made it this far!

15. Let the chocolate set up at room temperature for 30 minutes to 1 hour.

16. Using a brush, lightly tip the brush into the gold dust, if desired. Continue to lightly brush and blend the gold dust on top of the cereal treats, getting good coverage across the entire top of the treat. It's time to practice your blending.

17. Cover and store any leftover treats at room temperature for up to 3 days. To store, place in layers between sheets of parchment or wax paper.

RESOURCES & WORKS CITED

Beverage Recipes
Angostura bitters
Batiste Silver Rum
Bullet Rye Whiskey
Cointreau Liqueur
Everclear (120 proof)
Jinro Soju
Loco Tequila Blanco
Three Sheets Spiced Rum

Cannabis Flower
Aloha Humboldt
Alpenglow Farms
Moon Made Farms
Permanent Holiday

Concentrates
Aloha Humboldt Bubble Hash
Farmer & The Felon Papaya Punch
Kalya Extracts

Fresh Flower Cuttings
Hidden Farms x Permanent Holiday

Food Recipes
Du Four Classic Puff Pastry
Fly by Jing Chilis
Green Jay Gourmet Guava Jam
Gold Longevity Condensed Milk
Kara Coconut Cream
Red Boat Fish Sauce
San-J Tamari Gluten Free Soy Sauce

Gourmet Pantry Items
Dose of Saucy
Humboldt Sugar Co.
Pot d'Huile
Potli

Infusion/Decarboxylation Devices
Ardent FX decarboxylation & infusion device
LEVO II infusion device

Juices & Other Mixers
Coco Lopez Real Cream of Coconut
Dole 100% Pineapple Juice (not from concentrate)
Simply Lemonade (not from concentrate)
Twisted Alchemy Cold Pressed Juices (Passion Fruit and Blood Orange Juice)

Tinctures
Proof Wellness

WORKS CITED

Cannabis Spatula LLC. "Cannabis Dosage Calculator." Cannabis Spatula LLC, 2023.

Editor of Reader's Digest & Project CBD. "CBD & the Endocannabinoid System." Project CBD. September 2022.

Evans, J. *Cannabis Drinks: Secrets to Crafting CBD and THC Beverages at Home.* Fair Winds Press of Quarto Publishing Group, 2021.

Evans, J. *The Ultimate Guide to CBD: Explore the World of Cannabidiol.* Fair Winds Press of Quarto Publishing Group, 2020.

Goldleaf Ltd. *The Cooking Journal: A Cannabis Culinary Companion.* Fairfield, OH: Goldleaf Ltd., 2018.

Korkidis, John. "Fat-Washed Cannabis-Infused Alcohol." Chron Vivant. December 29, 2017.

Lee, Martin A. "Cannabis Dosing 101." Project CBD. May 2018.

Lee, Martin A. "The Endocannabinoid System." Project CBD.

Lee, Martin A. "Terpenes and the 'Entourage Effect.'" Project CBD.

Leinow, L., et al. *CBD: A Patient's Guide to Medicinal Cannabis.* Berkeley, CA: North Atlantic Books, 2018.

Lo, M. *The Weed Gummies Cookbook.* Ulysses Press, 2022.

Magner, E. "What Really Happens When You Mix CBD and Alcohol." Well+Good. September 28, 2019.

McDonough, E. "Top Tips for Using Hash as a Culinary Ingredient." Leafly. September 2018.

Mudge E. M., et al. "The Terroir of Cannabis: Terpene Metabolomics as a Tool to Understand Cannabis sativa Selections." Planta Medica. July 2019.

Ross, Michelle N. *Vitamin Weed: A 4-Step Plan to Prevent and Reverse Endocannabinoid Deficiency.* Green Stone Books, 2018.

Russo, Ethan. "Taming THC: Potential Cannabis Synergy and Phytocannabinoid-Terpenoid Entourage Effects." British Journal of Pharmacology. August 2011.

Staff Writer. "11-Hydroxy-THC—Increased Potency that Explains the Effect of Edibles?" Prof of Pot. July 2, 2019.

ABOUT THE AUTHORS

Haejin Chun

Haejin Chun is the founder, chef, and creative behind Big Bad Wolf SF. Establishing her culinary business in 2015, she is a first-generation Korean American chef, raised by immigrants. Following her passion, she has redefined the narrative of a first-generation Asian woman, cultivating independence and demonstrating the power of resilient hard work. She graduated from the California College of the Arts with a fine arts degree and a primary focus on installations, creating site-specific experiences and conceptually transformative spaces with skill sets that carry over to her events and set them apart from any normal dining experience.

Cannabis has been a part of Chun's life for the last two decades. Growing up in California, it was a lifestyle. Unknowingly, she's been creating culture and helping to normalize cannabis use since before legalization. Once California went recreational in 2018, it naturally opened the door and accelerated Chun's professional path into the cannabis industry. Building community and advocating for cannabis through positive representation has been her focus via her underground dinners and events company, Big Bad Wolf SF. She has also cultivated numerous brand partnerships and participated in educational panels. She was recognized nationally as a cannabis expert and consultant on Food Network's Chopped 420 TV show. Chun has been featured in articles in the *San Francisco Chronicle*, *High Times* magazine, *Leaf* magazine, Thrillist, Eater, and KQED among many others.

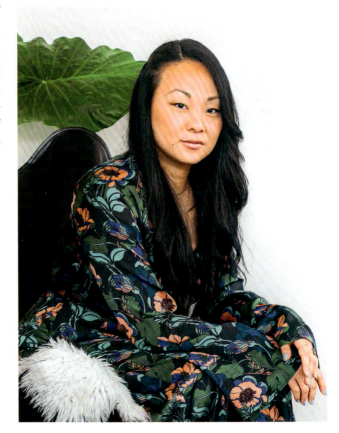

Currently, Chun is focusing on a members-only, private cannabis supper club for women in San Francisco via her branch off, Big Bad Queens, a safe space to break bread together, combined with the ritual and ceremony of cannabis while cultivating community. Follow Chef Haejin Chun and Big Bad Wolf SF on Instagram @bigbadwolfsf.

Jamie Evans

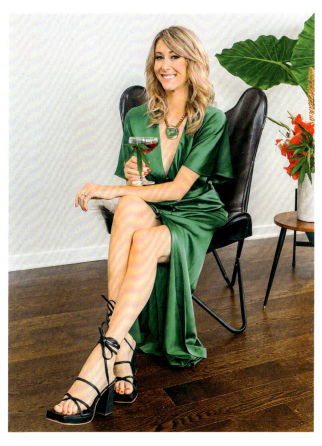

Jamie Evans is the founder of The Herb Somm, a culinary-meets-cannabis blog and lifestyle brand that's focused on the gourmet side of the cannabis industry. She's an author, entrepreneur, and writer specializing in cannabis, beverages, food, wine, and the canna-culinary world.

As a well-known cannabis and wine personality, Jamie is best known for her literary work and signature canna-culinary events. She's contributed to POPSUGAR, Wine Enthusiast magazine, High Times magazine, MARY magazine, and The Clever Root magazine specializing in lifestyle features for the modern consumer. She's the co-editor of GoldLeaf's acclaimed cannabis cooking journal and published author of the books The Ultimate Guide to CBD: Explore the World of Cannabidiol (Fair Winds Press, 2020) and Cannabis Drinks: Secrets to Crafting CBD and THC Beverages at Home (Fair Winds Press, 2021).

As an industry leader, Jamie was named as one of Wine Enthusiast Magazine's Top 40 Under 40 Tastemakers in 2018 and as a 2018 Innovator by SevenFifty Daily. She was also recognized as one of Green Market Report's "Most Important Women in Weed" in 2020 and named as one of Marijuana Venture's Top 40 Under 40 leaders in 2023.

Alongside her work in the cannabis space, Jamie is a Certified Sommelier with over a decade of wine industry experience. She's been featured in dozens of different articles and TV segments, including Food & Wine, Wall Street Journal, Entrepreneur, Forbes, Financial Times, Wine Enthusiast, Robb Report, San Francisco Chronicle, Los Angeles Times, ABC, and High Times, among many others. Follow Jamie's canna-culinary adventures on Instagram @theherbsomm.

ACKNOWLEDGMENTS

This book was truly a team effort! First, we'd like to thank our publisher, Insight Editions, and our licensor, High Times, for this incredible opportunity and for supporting our vision.

We'd also like to thank our wonderful editor, Sammy Holland, editorial assistant, Emma Merwin, and creative director, Chrissy Kwasnik. We couldn't have done this without you!

We are also so grateful to have had the opportunity to work with our legendary photographer, Eva Kolenko and Our House Studio based in Petaluma. A big shout out and thank you to Eva, our fantastic food stylist, Natalie Drobny, photo studio manager and assistant, Genesis Vallejo, and onsite chefs, Michael Andreatta and Huxley McCorkle. This book is absolutely stunning, thanks to you. Cheers!

A heartfelt thank you to our expert contributors and canna-friends Nicole Dimascio, Vince Bugtong, Mennlay Golokeh Aggrey, Manny Mendoza, Wendy Zeng, Monica Lo, and Christopher Jacob. Thank you for all your work in this space and for pushing the boundaries in the kitchen.

Finally, so much gratitude to all of the cannabis trailblazers, activists, and pioneers who have paved the way. We are forever grateful for your passion, perseverance, and endless commitment to the cannabis plant.

Haejin Chun

All my love to my grandmother who cooked for me almost every day from when I was in the womb until I was ready to leave for college for always placing something yummy on top of my tiny spoonful of rice, every time baby Haejin held it out for her. She inspired most of these recipes. I'm thankful to my mom who did her best as a single mother to put food on the table; it was her sacrifices and hard work that afforded me the privileges to access the opportunities she never had. And to my late grandfather who gave me my voice, that loud and proud, fight and fire in me.

I could not have written this book without my dear friend and co-author Jamie Evans. You truly are an expert in your purpose. I've learned so much from you during this process, not just about bookmaking but about being a gracious, supportive, and solid human being in general. Thank you for everything.

To my bestie, Leslie Yoon, who has always been there for me for all the good and bad. The only other person that really knows who I was and everything it took to get to the person I am today. You gave meaning to finding my chosen family. Thank you for being a constant source of comfort and laughs. I would be a puddle on the floor without you . . . until the wheels fall off.

Thankful for my partner, Marc Flynn, who was my rock every time I started doubting myself or my recipes while writing this book. Thank you for always encouraging me to shine brighter and being the type of man that can stand proudly next to a strong woman. You've loved me through it all. Your knowledge and passion in the cannabis industry has been an endless resource for me. We've been building together from our mutual love for weed since day one.

To my pup and baby girl, Rye, thank you for patiently waiting for something to drop on the floor during recipe testing and enthusiastically eating it up like it was the most delicious morsel that ever existed.

I'm grateful for every single person that came before me who helped advocate to normalize cannabis. I'm especially thankful for friends like Monica Lo (@sousweed), Tess Melody (@tessmelody), Hilary Yu (@ouracademy), Lulu Tsui (@ontherevel), and Tammy Pettigrew (@thecannabiscutie) to name a few, for being fierce women in the industry and who I deeply admire in their efforts to educate and push boundaries with so much heart. To everyone who continues to bring so much value and a sense of community to the industry, thank you.

To anyone who's ever believed in me, cheered me on, come to one of my events, said "yes," spoken my name in a room of opportunities, made me feel seen, or mirrored back my gestures as an affirmation . . . I would not be here without you. You have been fuel for my journey and it has been the greatest gift I've ever received. Thank you from the deepest places of everything that I am.

Jamie Evans

A heartfelt thank you to my grandparents for instilling my passion for food! I also want to thank my amazing co-author, Haejin Chun. It's been such an honor and dream to be on this journey with you. Cheers to the beautiful book baby we created. Love you!

I am so grateful for my mother, who passed away in 2019. She knew how to live life to the fullest and always encouraged me to follow my dreams. I am also so grateful for my father, who has always been there for me and has supported my dreams since day one.

A major shout-out and heartfelt thank you to my wonderful husband, Stratos. You are truly my rock and soul mate! I wouldn't be where I am today without you. I also want to thank my sister, Kayla, and brother-in-law, Mishka, who have been The Herb Somm's number-one fans since the beginning! Thank you to my extended families, the Barbers, the Evanses, the Christianakises, and the vom Dorps, for your support and believing in my vision to write three cannabis books! I love you.

Last but not least, I want to thank my fantastic fans and readers who've continued to support my work. Much love and gratitude to all!

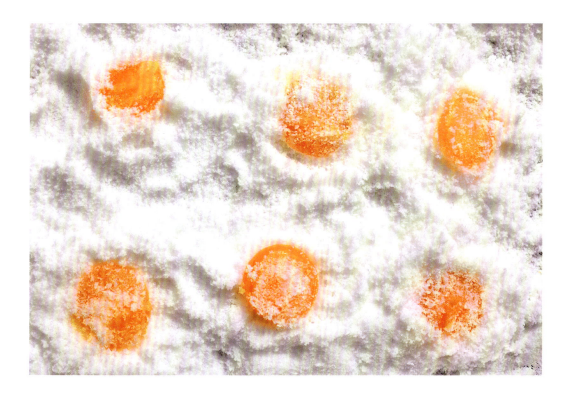

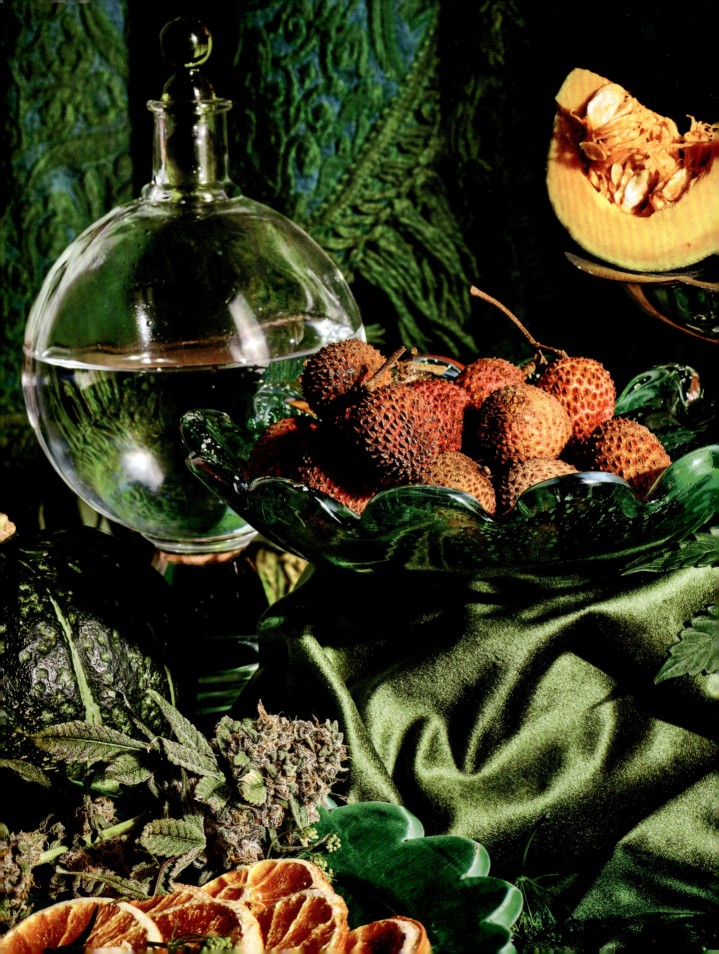

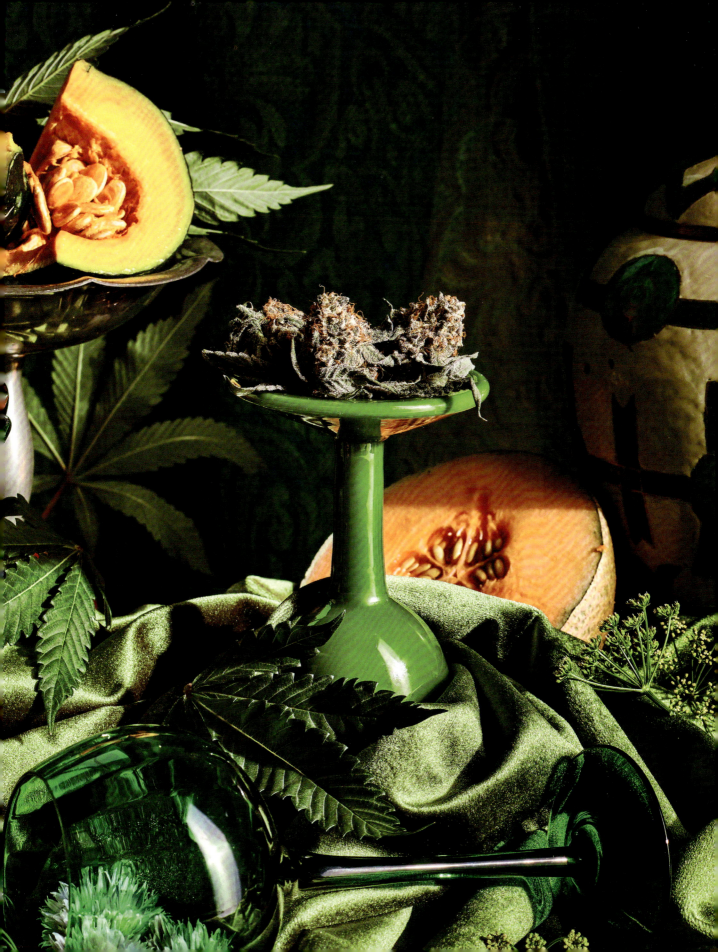

PO Box 3088
San Rafael, CA 94912
www.insighteditions.com

Find us on Facebook: www.facebook.com/InsightEditions
Follow us on Instagram: @insighteditions
Follow us on Twitter: @insighteditions

© High Times 2023

All rights reserved. Published by Insight Editions, San Rafael, California, in 2023.

No part of this book may be reproduced in any form without written permission from the publisher.

ISBN: 979-8-88663-189-0

Publisher: Raoul Goff
VP, Co-Publisher: Vanessa Lopez
VP, Creative: Chrissy Kwasnik
VP, Manufacturing: Alix Nicholaeff
VP, Group Managing Editor: Vicki Jaeger
Publishing Director: Jamie Thompson
Designer: Lola Villanueva
Senior Editor: Samantha Holland
Editorial Assistant: Emma Merwin
Managing Editor: Maria Spano
Senior Production Editor: Katie Rokakis
Production Associate: Deena Hashem
Senior Production Manager, Subsidiary Rights: Lina s Palma-Temena

Food Recipes © 2023 Haejin Chun
Drink Recipes © 2023 Jamie Evans
Author Headshot Photographer: Monica Lo

Photographer: Eva Kolenko
Photography Assistant: Genesis Vallejo
Food Stylist: Natalie Drobny
Food Assistants: Michael Andretta and Huxley McCorkle

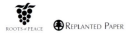

Insight Editions, in association with Roots of Peace, will plant two trees for each tree used in the manufacturing of this book. Roots of Peace is an internationally renowned humanitarian organization dedicated to eradicating land mines worldwide and converting war-torn lands into productive farms and wildlife habitats. Roots of Peace will plant two million fruit and nut trees in Afghanistan and provide farmers there with the skills and support necessary for sustainable land use.

Manufactured in China by Insight Editions

10 9 8 7 6 5 4 3 2 1

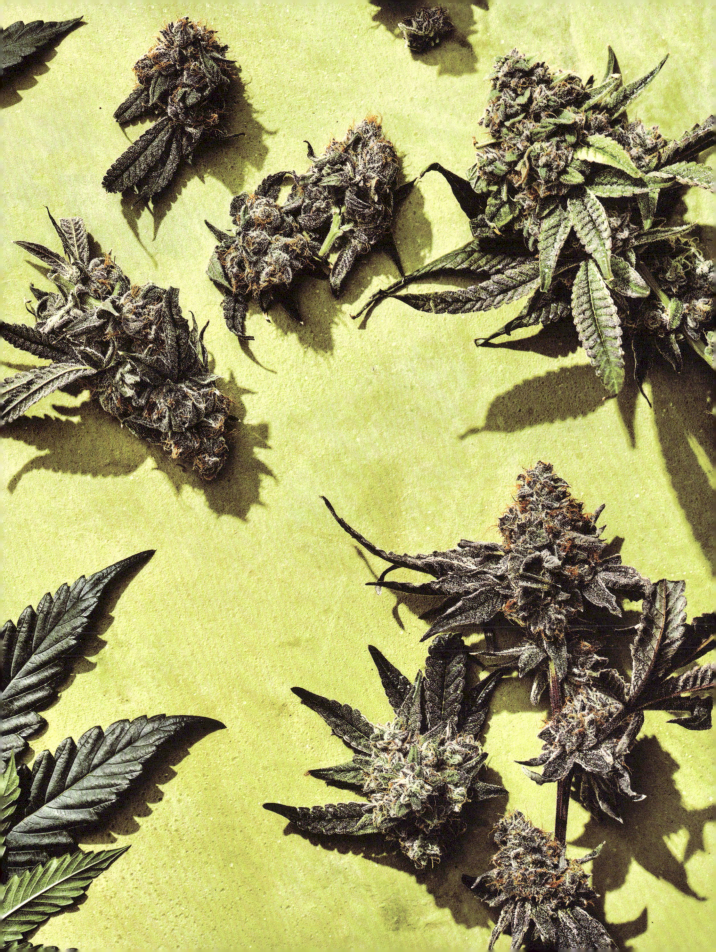

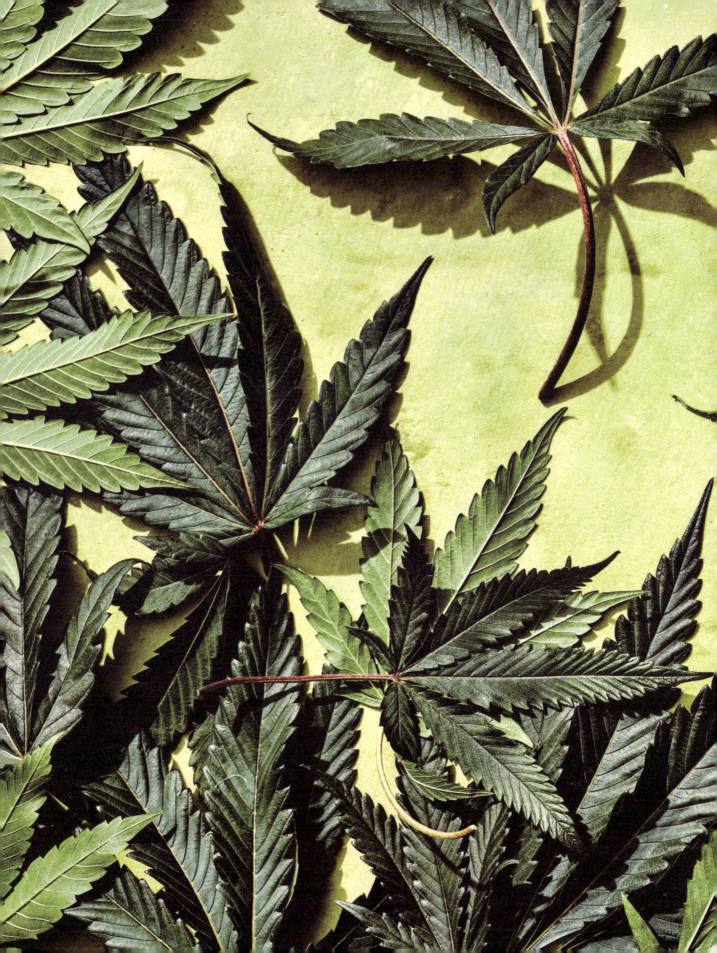